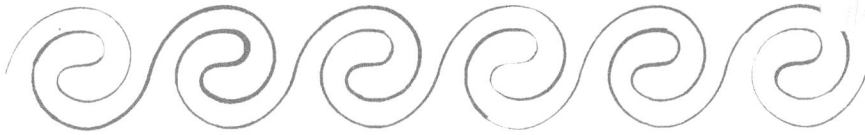

This Dental Health
Log Book
belongs to:

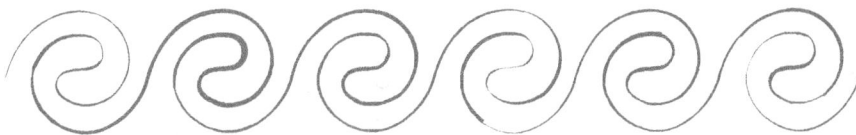

_____

_____

How to use this Dental Health Notebook:

This useful dental health planner is a must-have for anyone that needs to record their kids dental health activities! You will love this easy to use dental health log book to track and record all your dental health activities.

Each interior page includes space to record & track the following:

Draw pictures of the dentist - Record and have the kids draw pictures of the dentist.

Tooth Fairy Drawing - Use this space to draw a tooth fairy.

Reminder Page - Stay on task, have the kids say out loud the clean teeth affirmations.

Happy Tooth Drawing - Fill in this space, have the kids draw a happy tooth.

Dental Cleaning Appointments - Stay on task by writing down the dates of the next teeth cleaning.

Tooth Fairy Thank You Note - Record a note of thanks to the tooth fairy.

Coloring Pages - Dental themed coloring pages.

If you are new to taking kids to the dentist, or have been at it for a while this dental health log book is a must have! Can make a great useful gift for any parents teaching kids about the dentist!

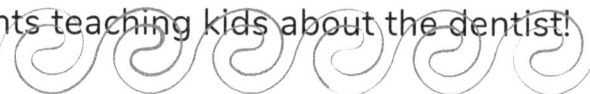

Enjoy!

Draw a picture of a tooth:

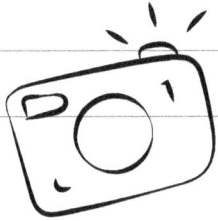

Draw a picture of your dentist

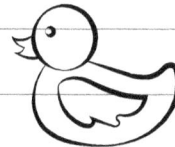

Draw a picture of your toothbrush:

Draw a picture of the tooth fairy:

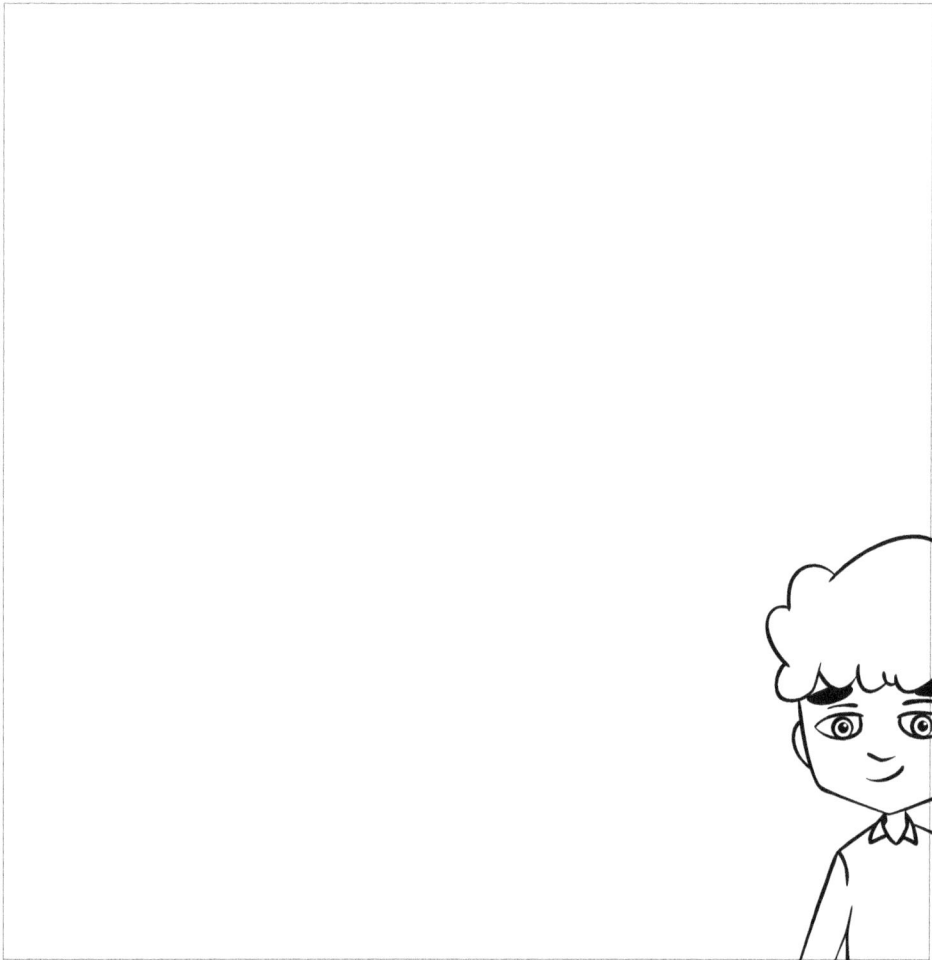

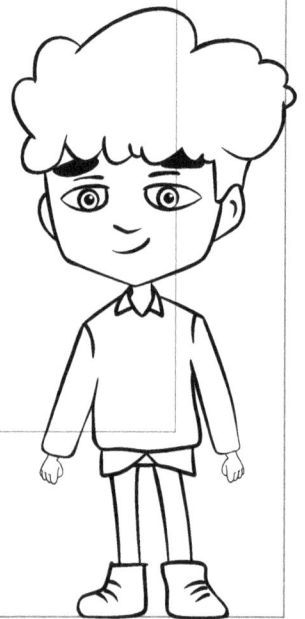

Date: _____

I can brush my teeth	I use a toothbrush
The dentist checks my teeth	My teeth are happy!

write a lil story about going to the dentist:

_____

_____

_____

Draw a picture of a happy tooth!

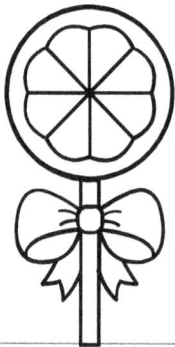

Draw a picture of dental floss:

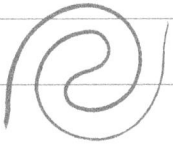

Draw a picture of the dental office:

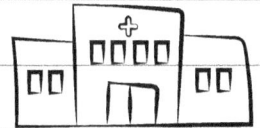

Draw a picture of the dental hygienist:

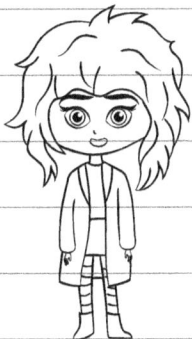

Date: _____

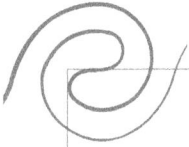

I will Floss my teeth everyday

Did I eat alot of sugar today?

How do my teeth feel today?

I will use mouthwash everyday

Write a lil story about your teeth:

_____

_____

_____

_____

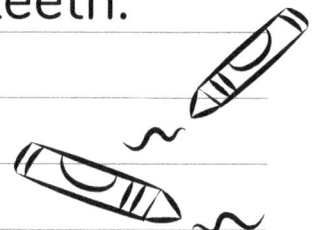

Date: _____

My Next Dental Cleaning Will Be:

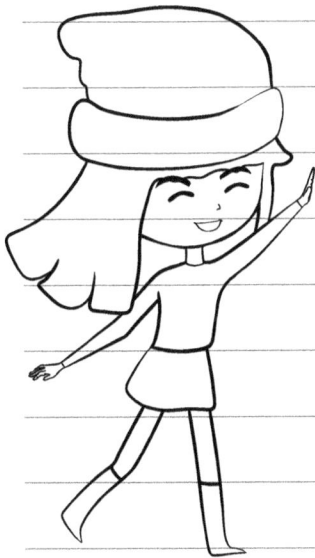

_____

_____

_____

_____

_____

_____

_____

_____

_____

_____

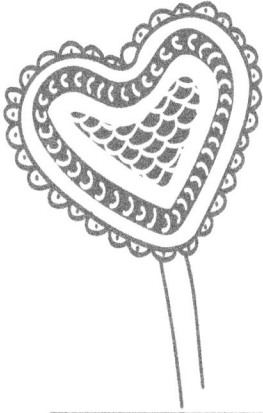

Write a note of thanks to the tooth fairy:

My tooth came out on this date

Write the amount the tooth fairy left
under your pillow

Practice Writing:

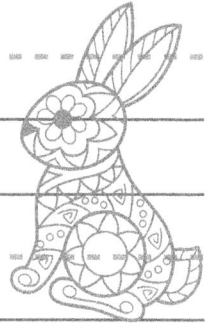

I have happy teeth

I love to brush my teeth

I love to floss my teeth

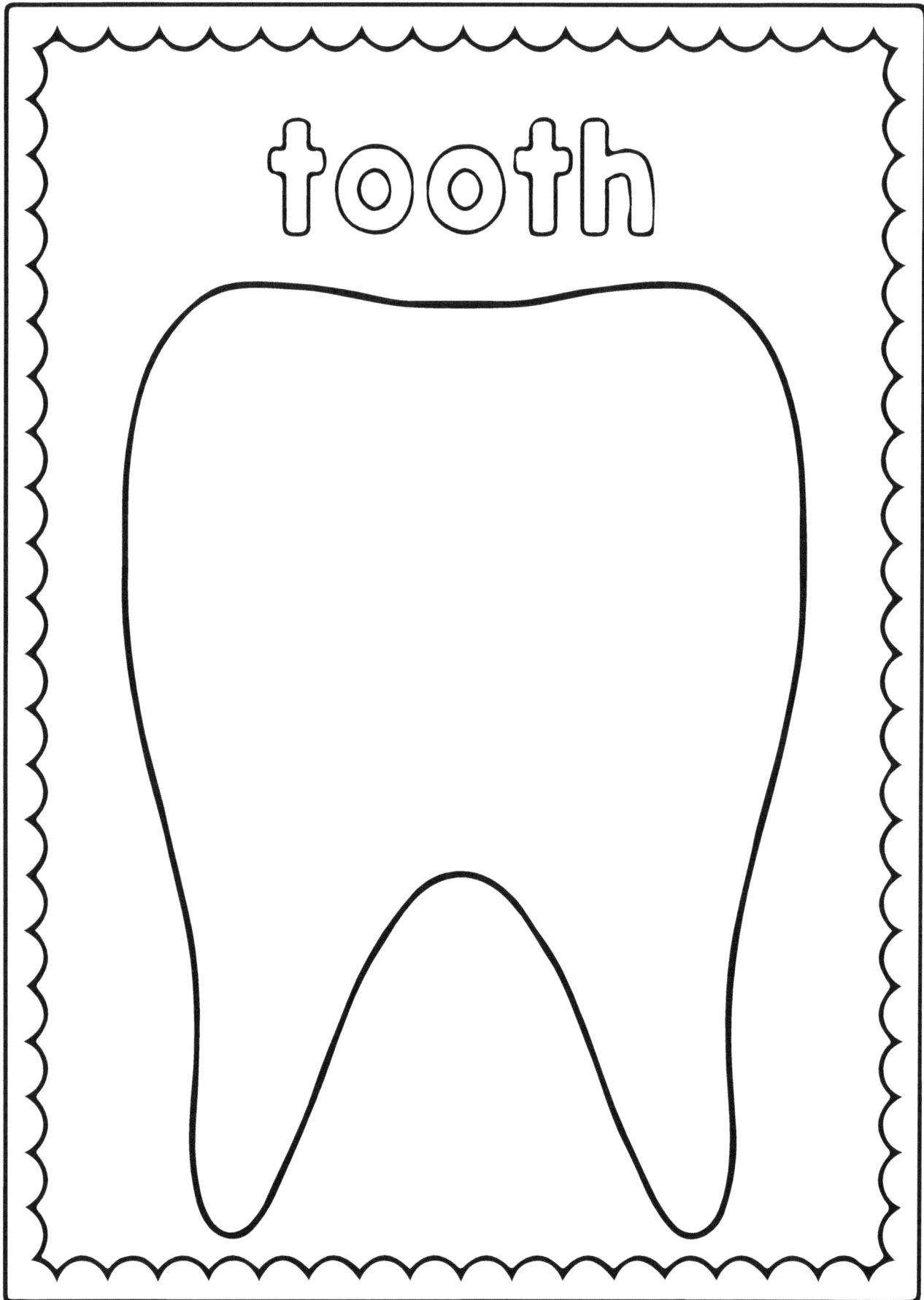

tooth

tooth x-ray

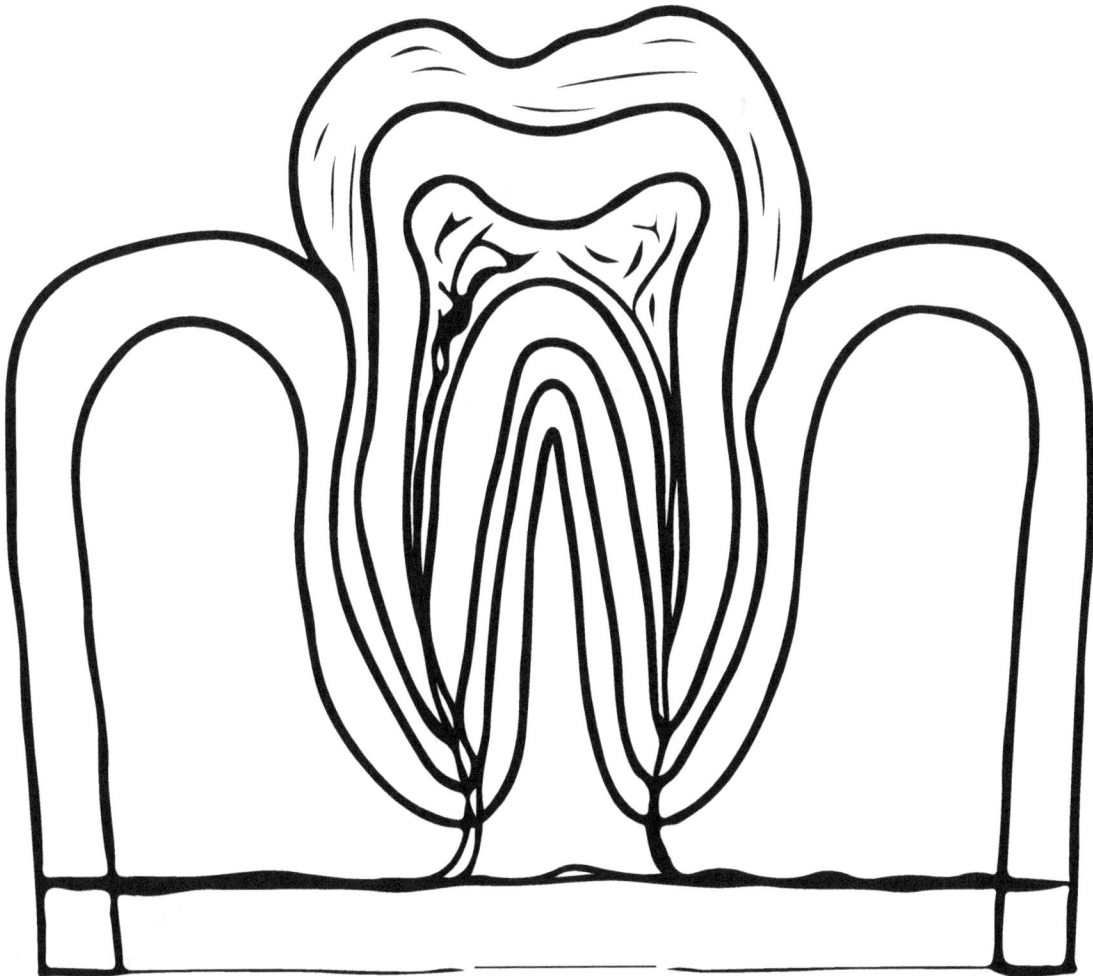

cavity

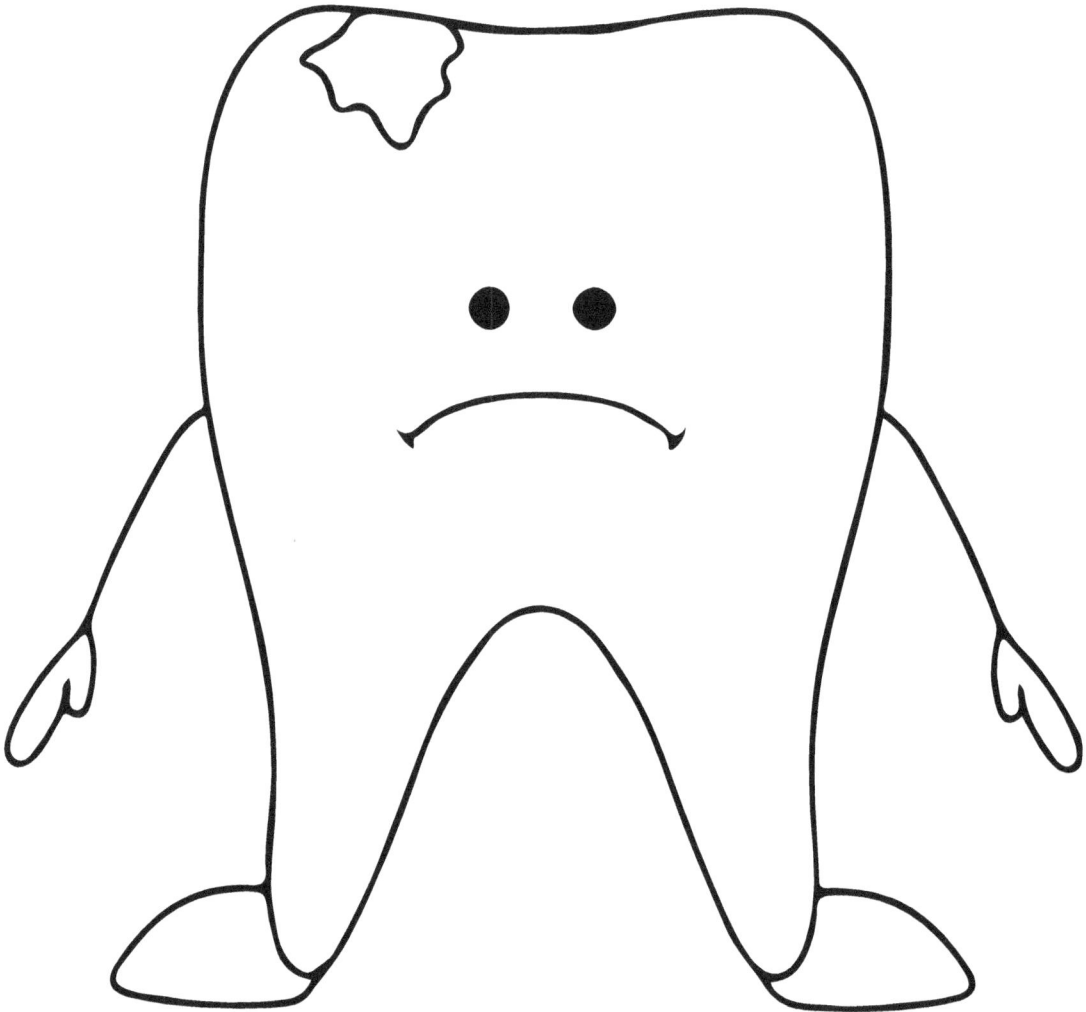

check-up

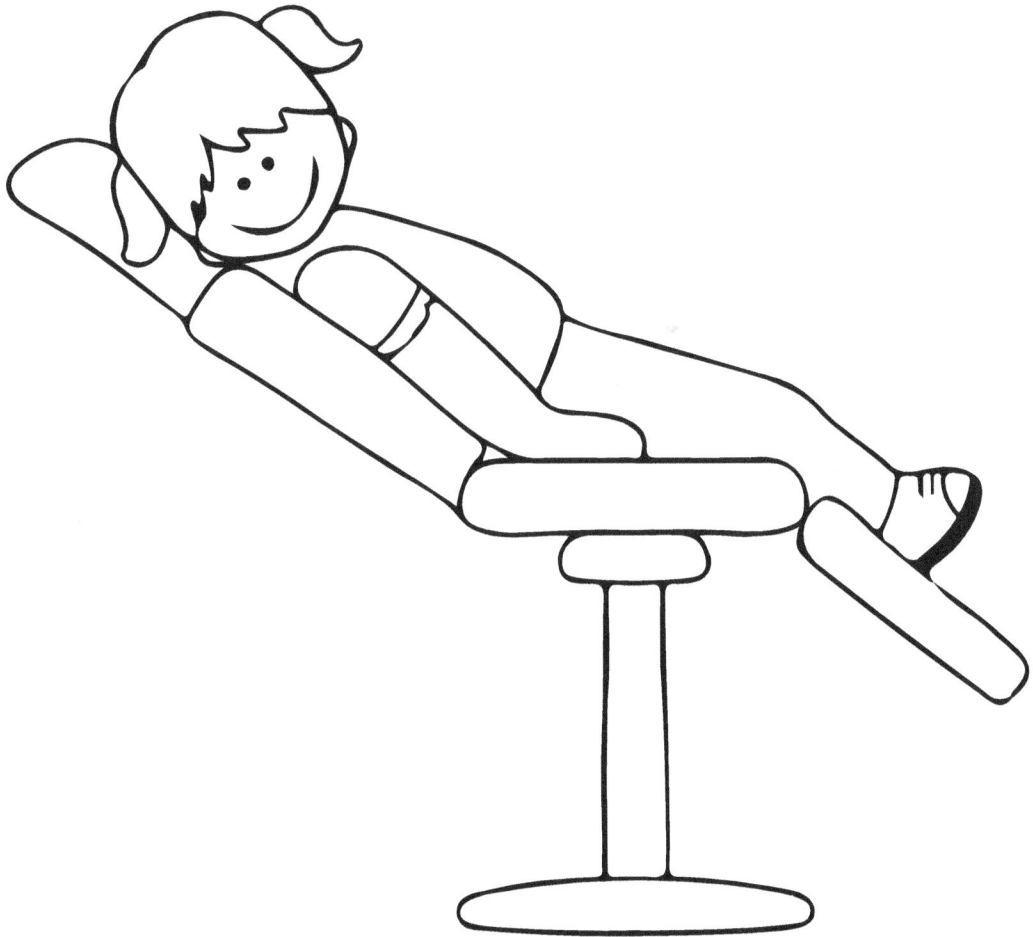

Tooth Fairy

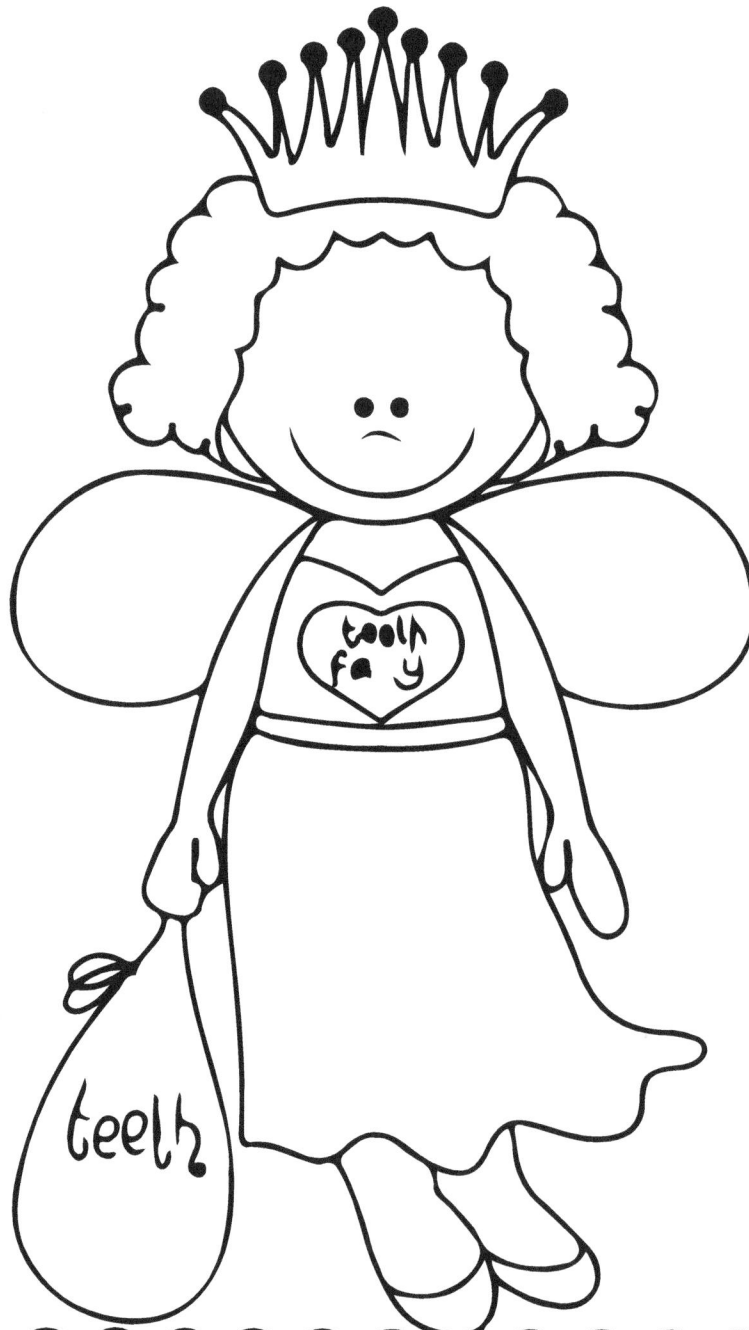

dentist

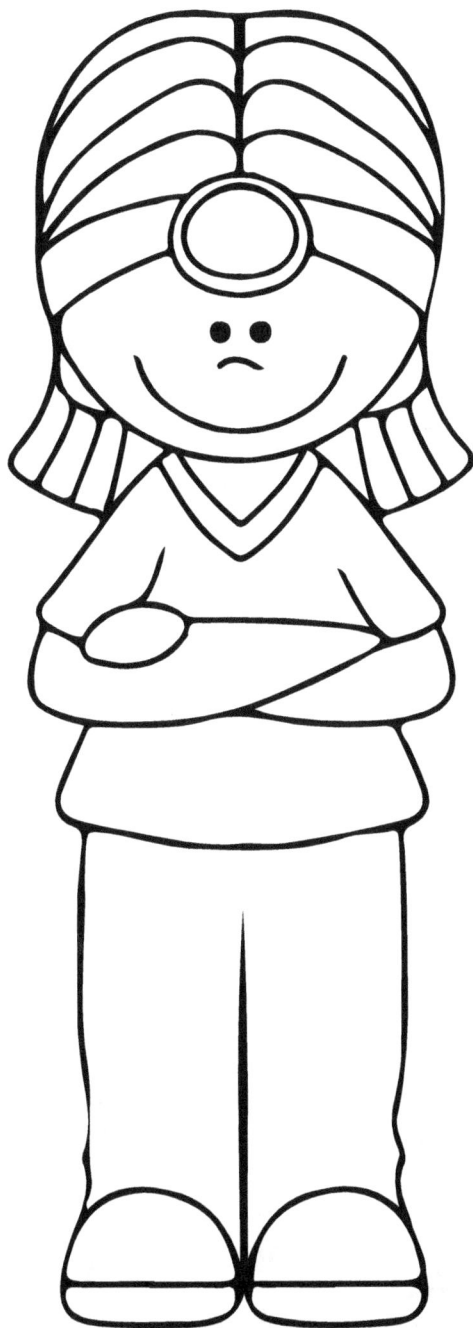

dentist

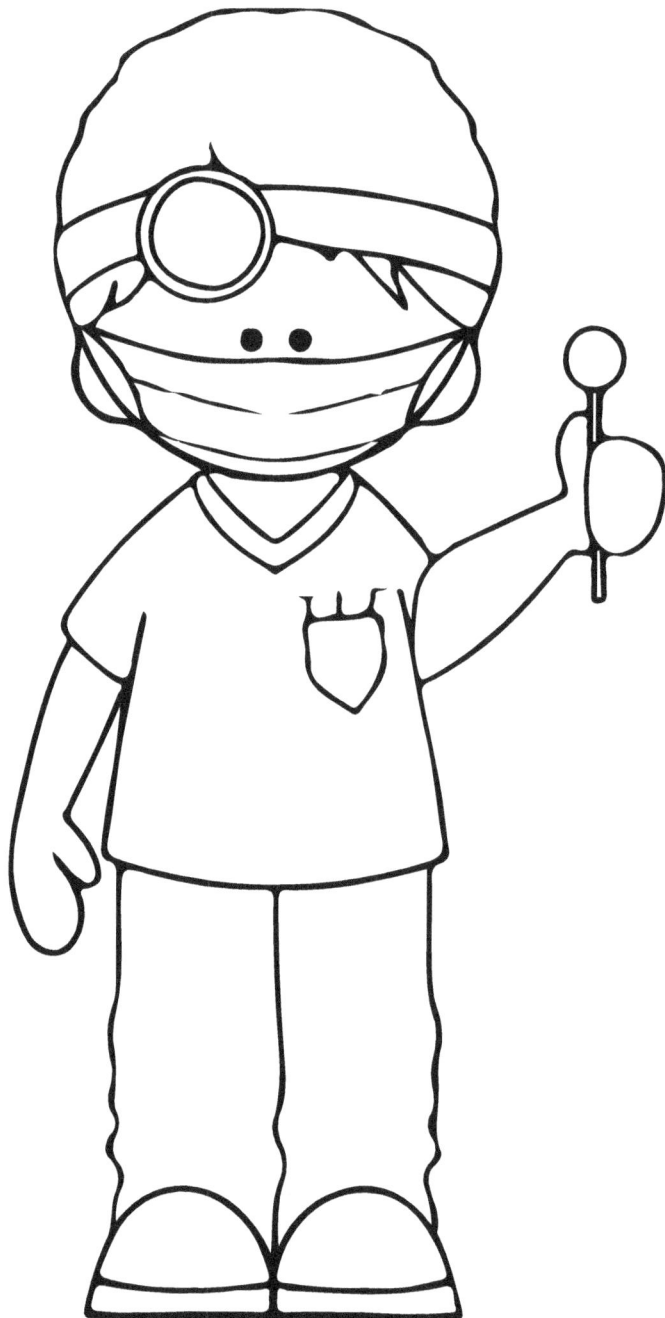

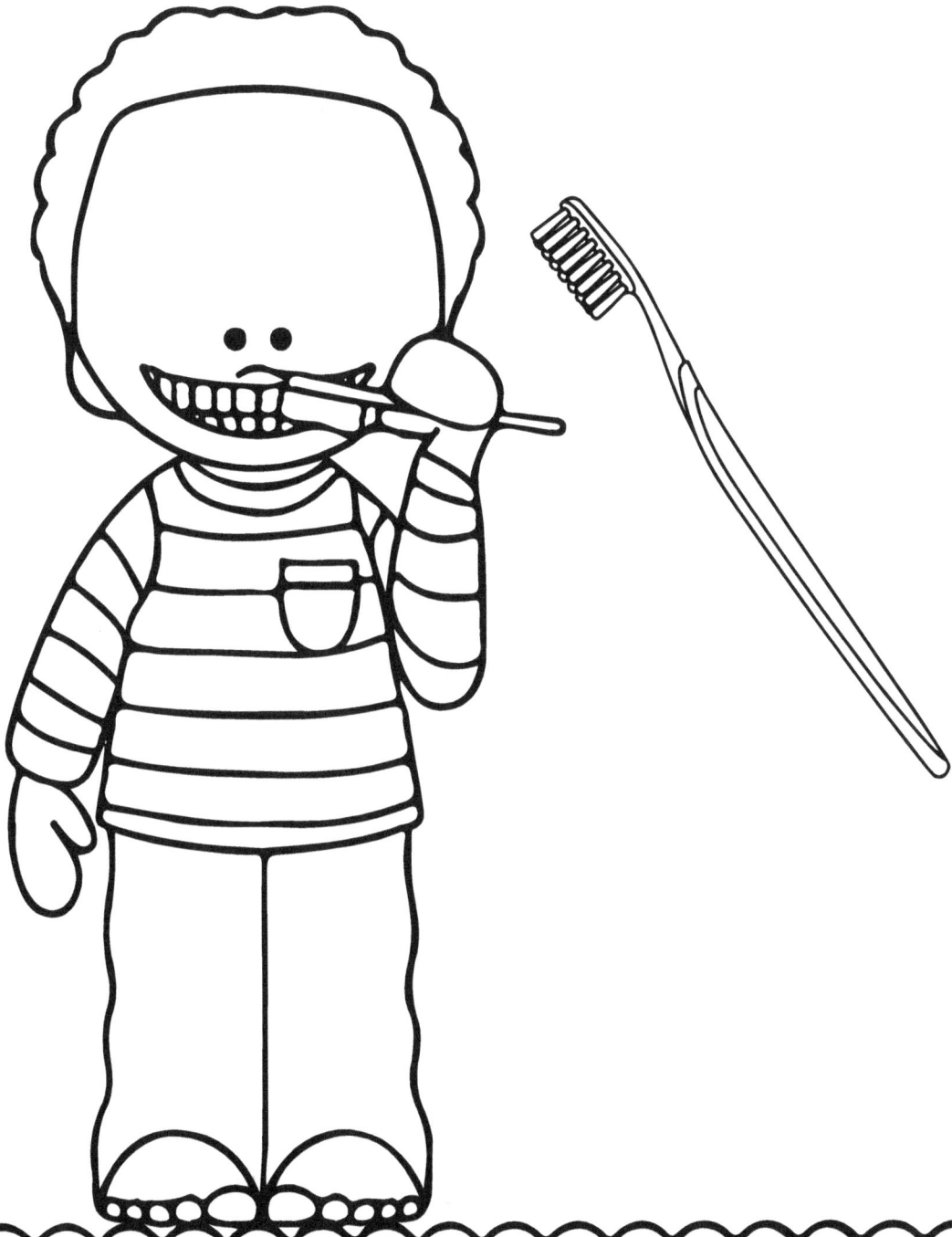

brush

brush

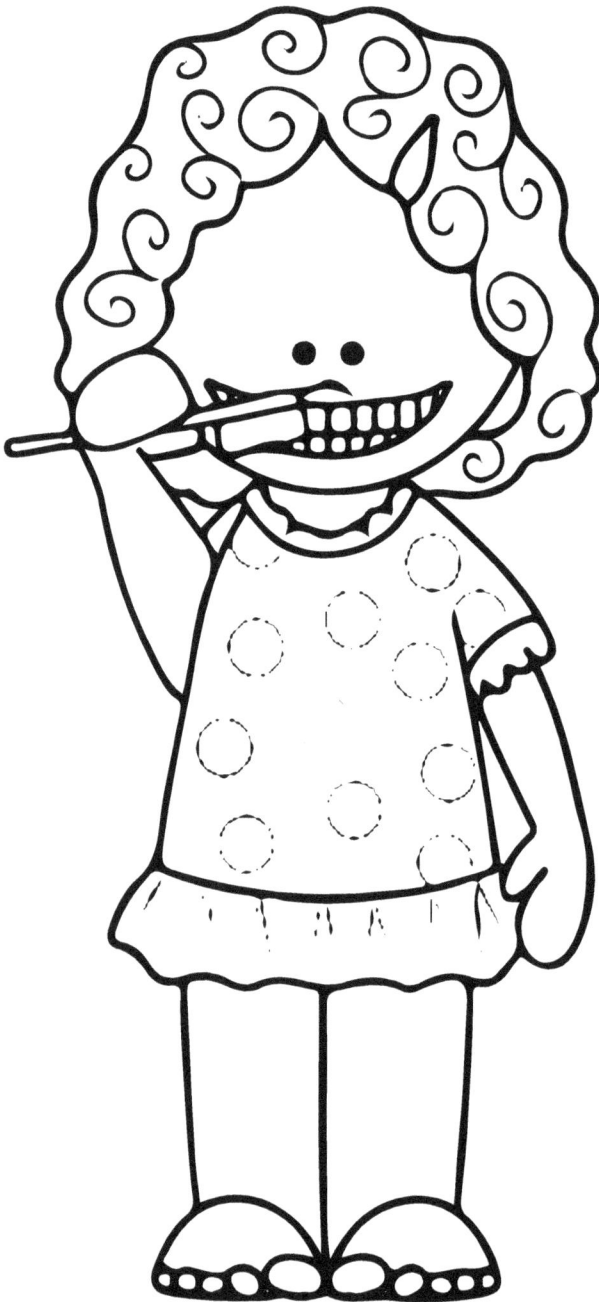
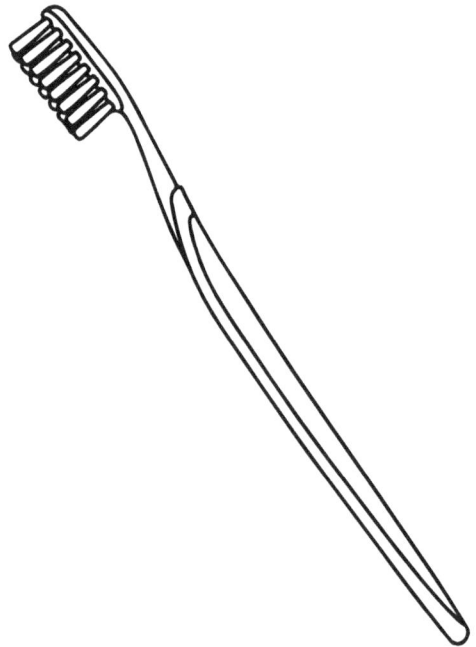

floss

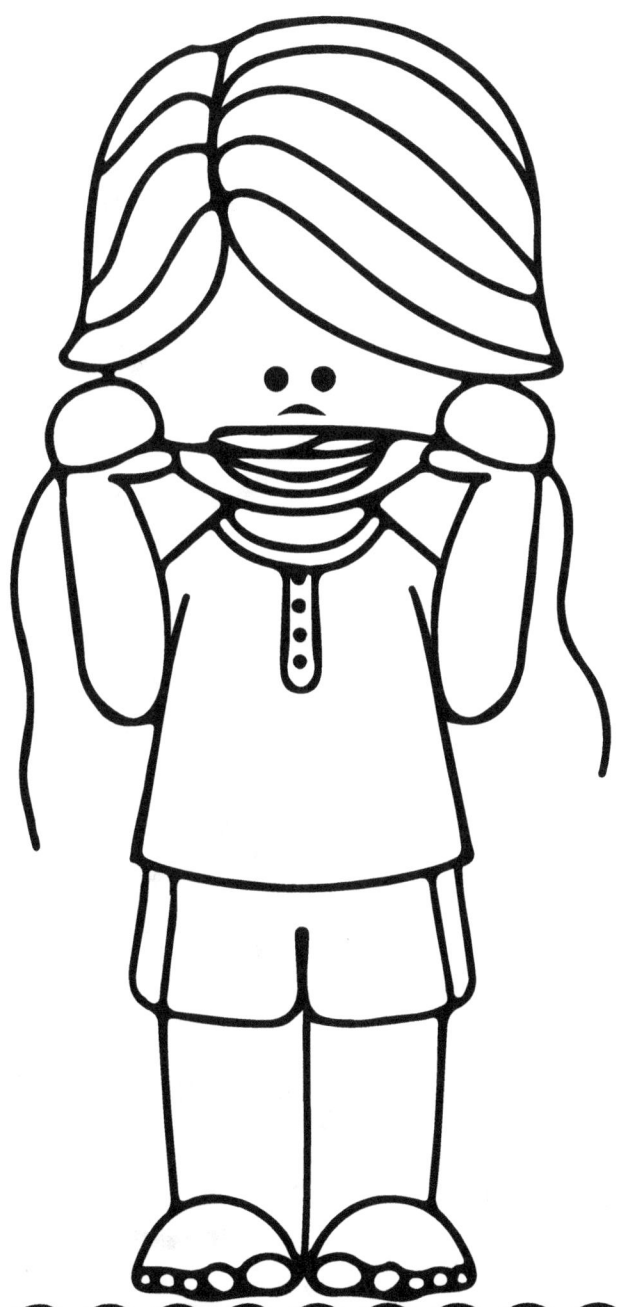

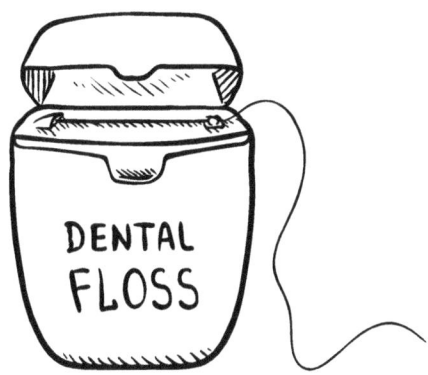

DENTAL FLOSS

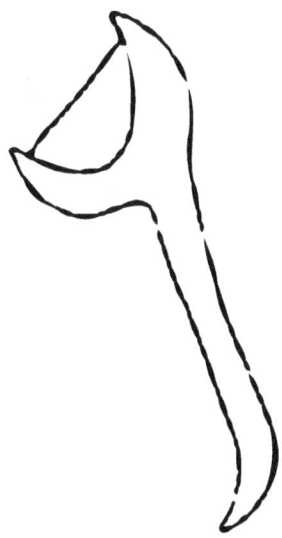

Color. Match.

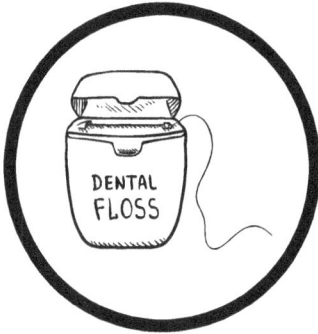

tooth

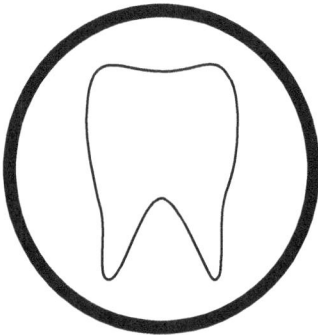

floss

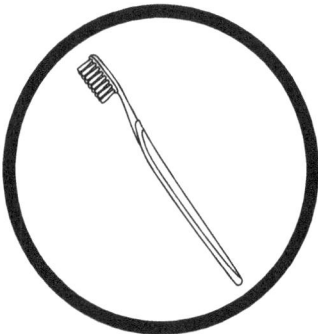

dentist

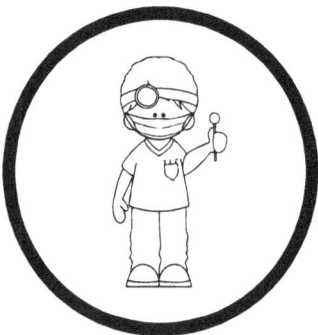

toothbrush

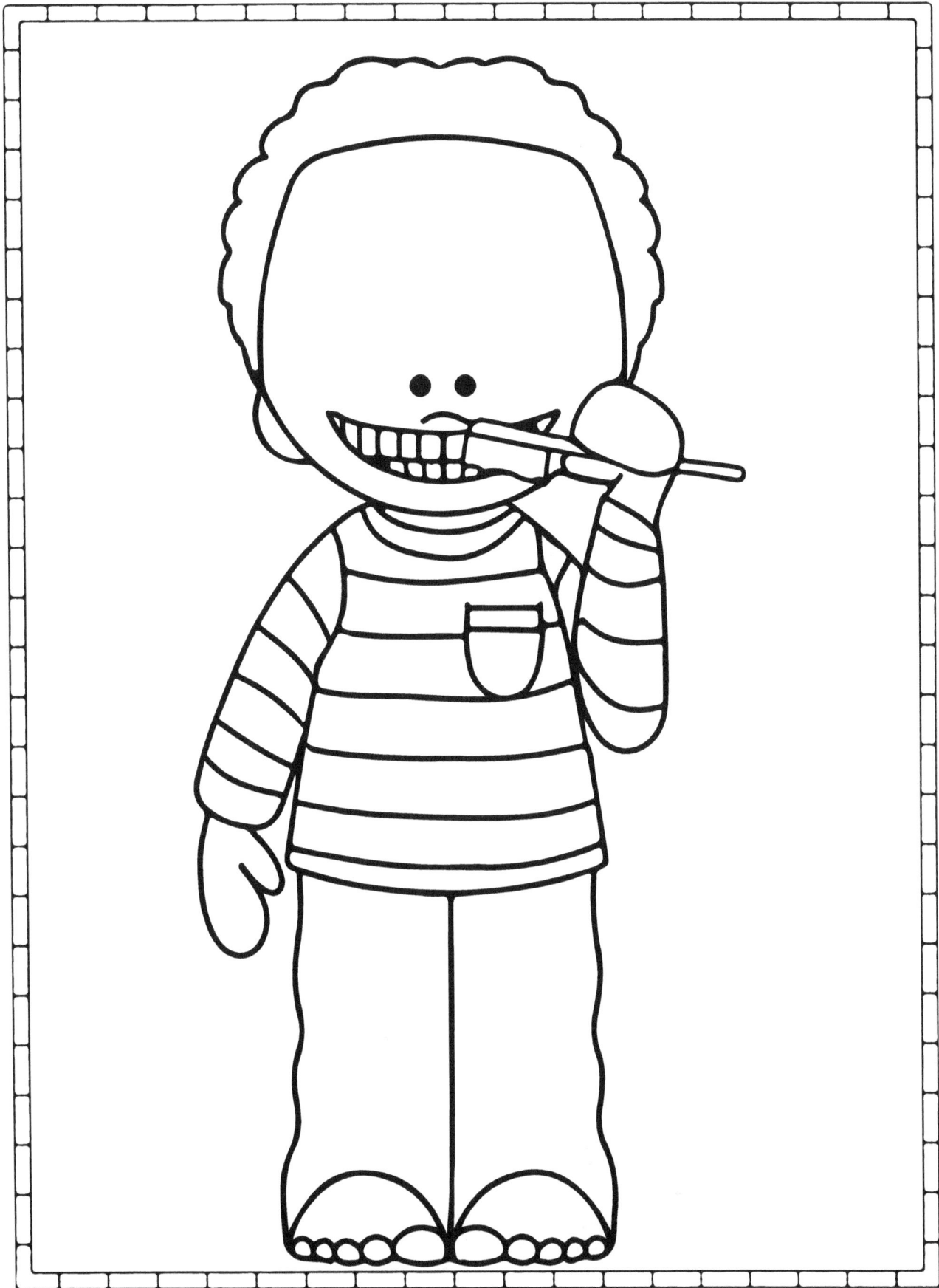

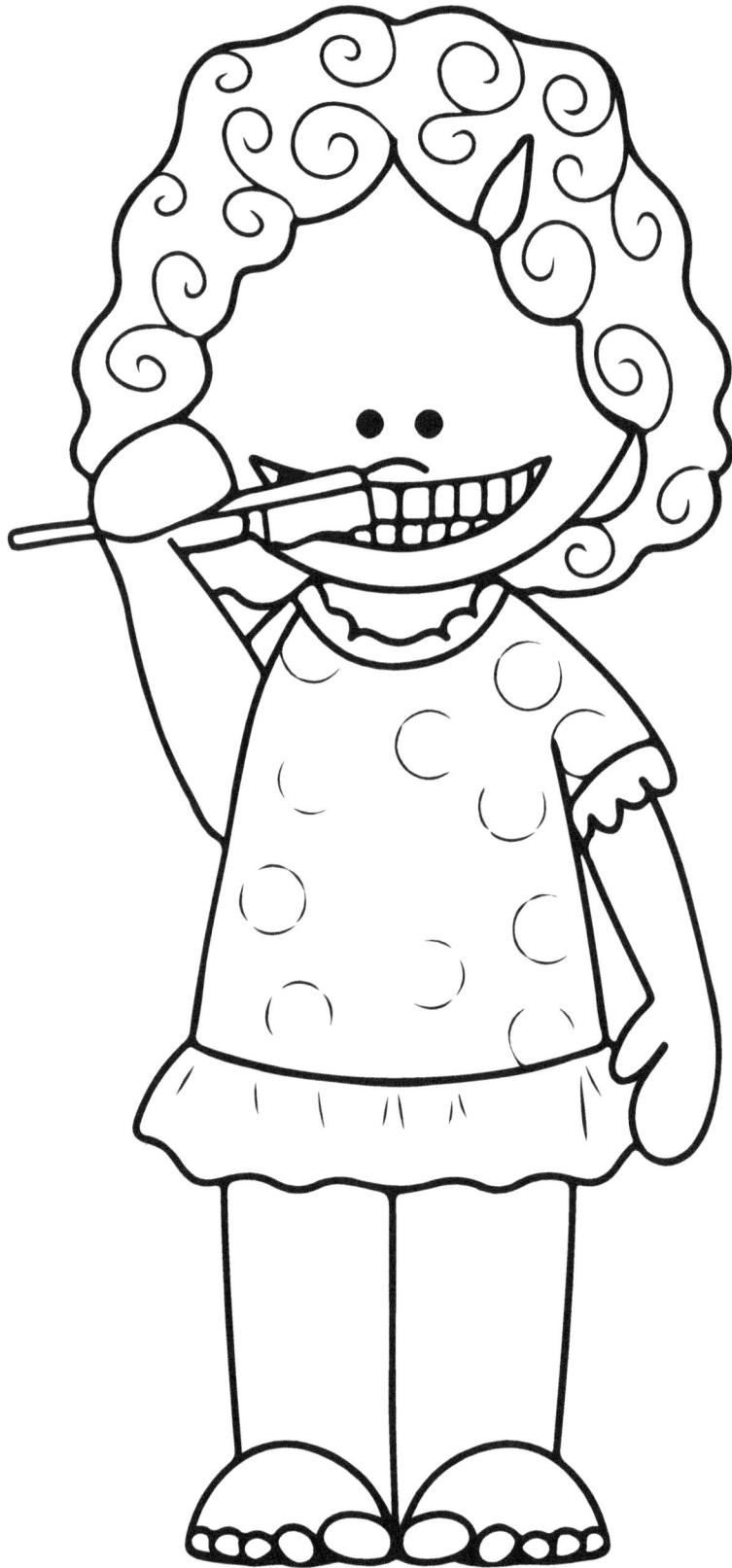

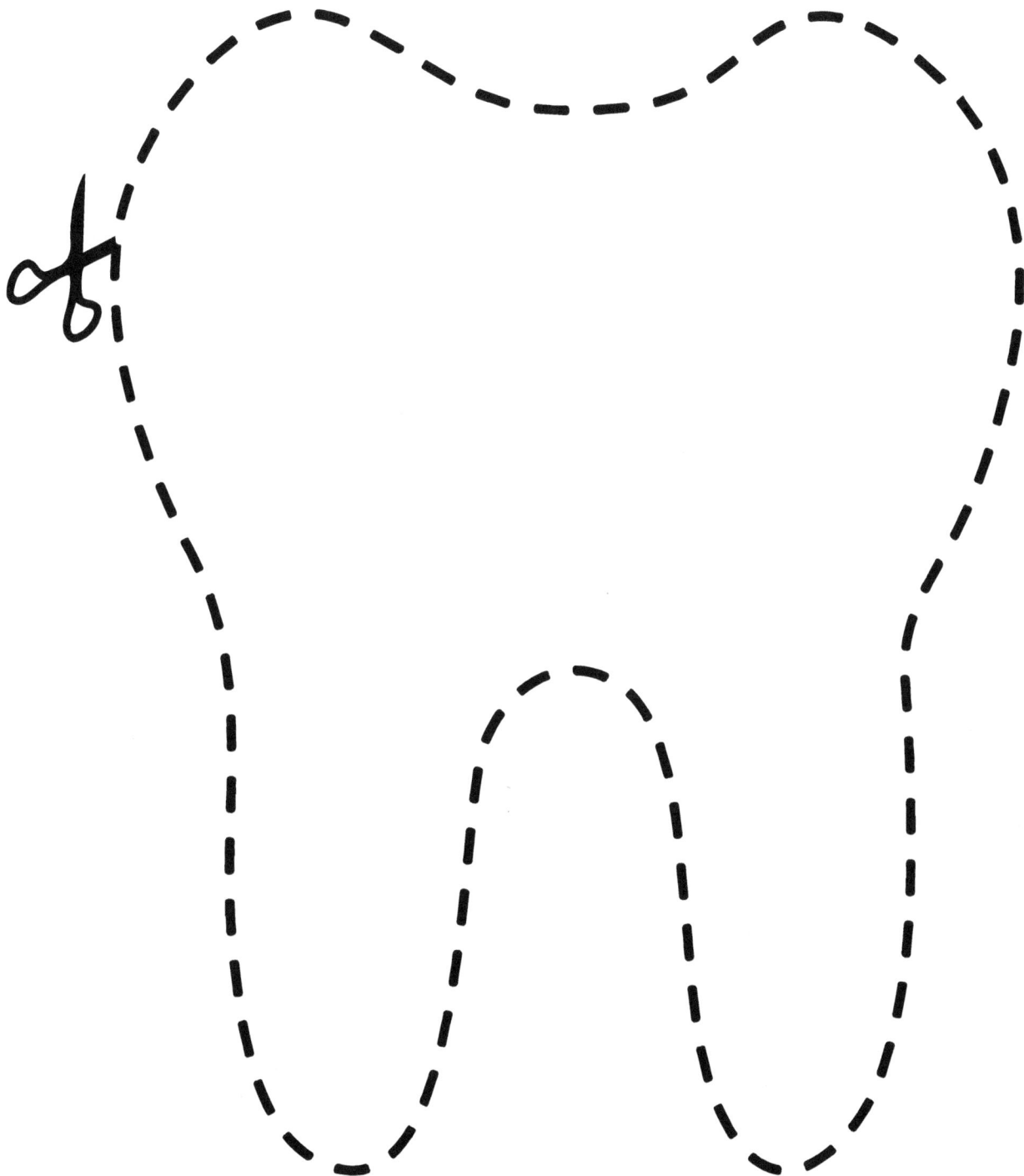

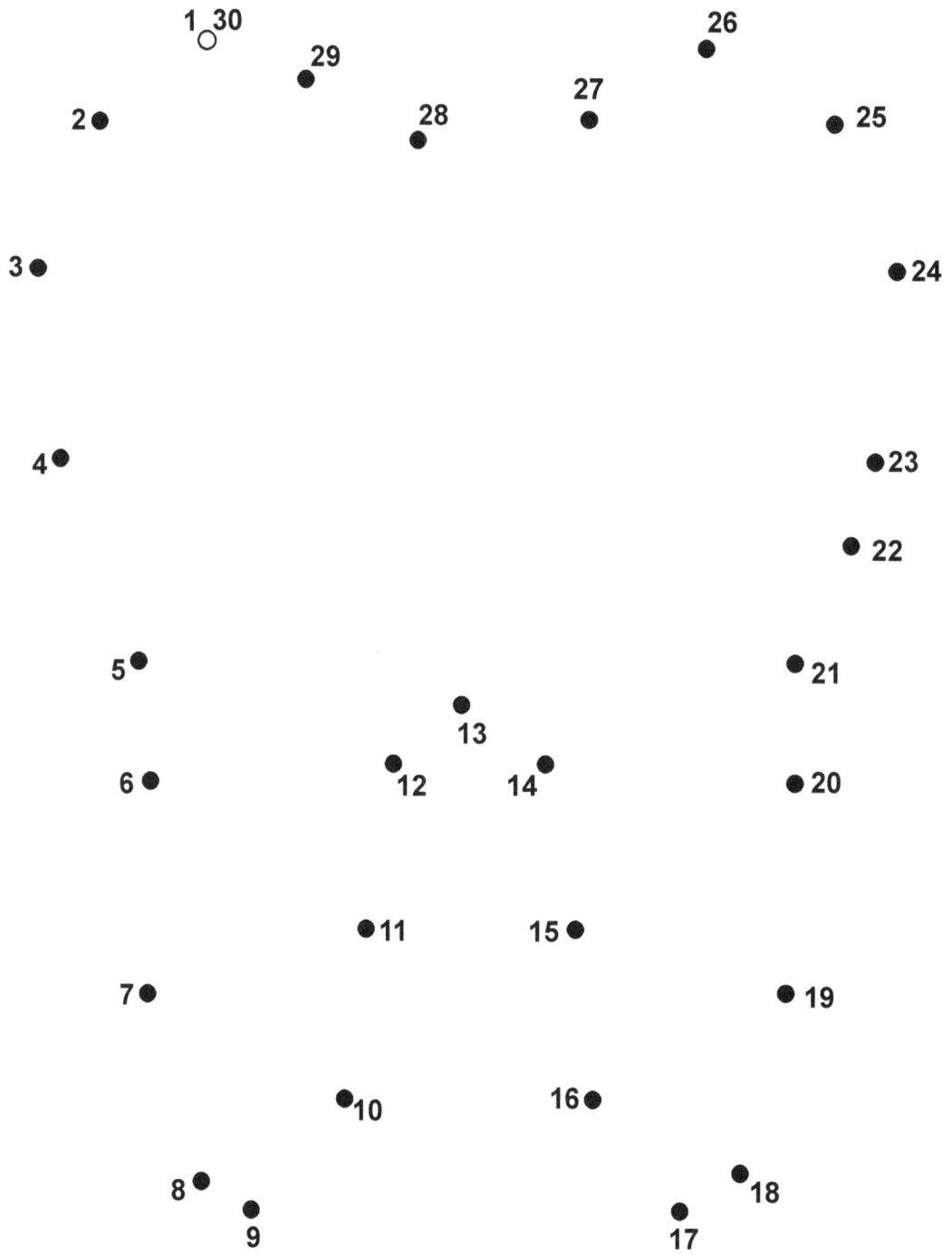

1 30

29

26

2

27

28

25

3

24

4

23

22

5

13

21

6

12

14

20

11

15

7

19

10

16

18

8

9

17

Draw a picture of a tooth:

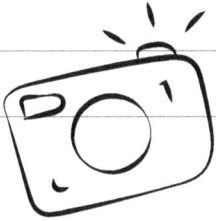

_____

_____

_____

_____

_____

Draw a picture of your dentist

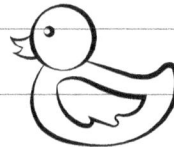

_____

_____

_____

_____

Draw a picture of your toothbrush:

_____

_____

_____

_____

_____

Draw a picture of the tooth fairy:

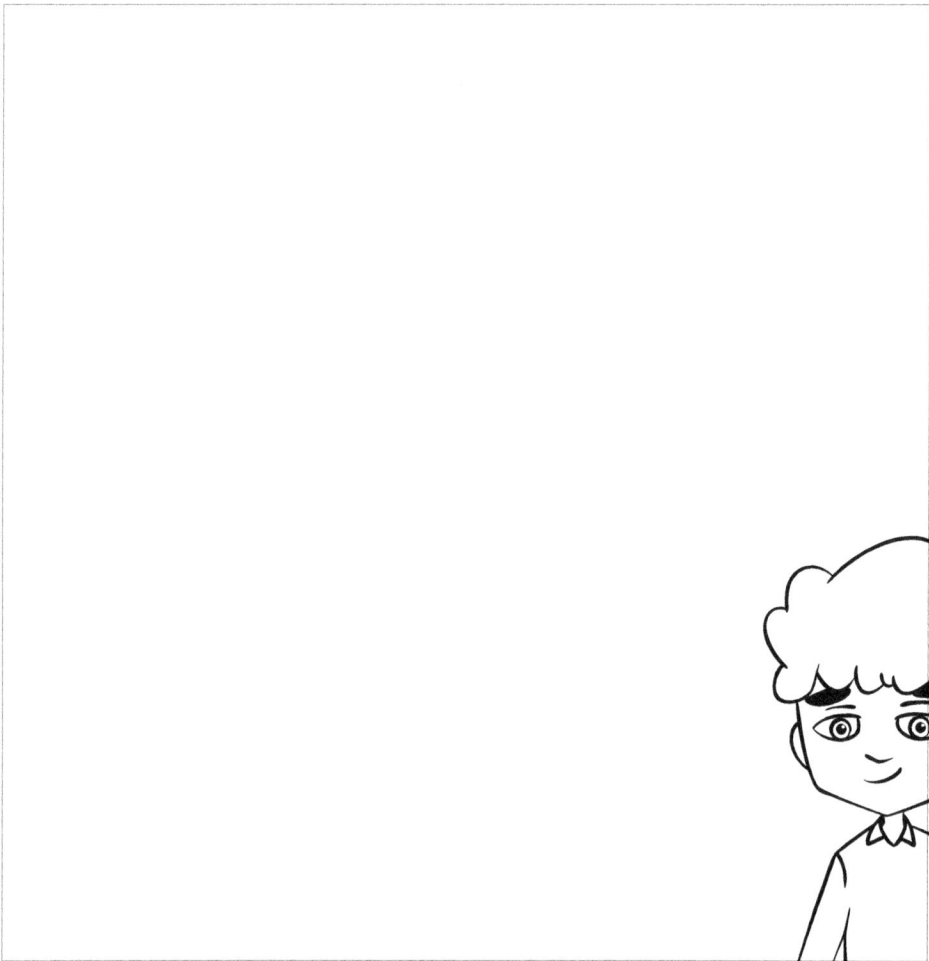

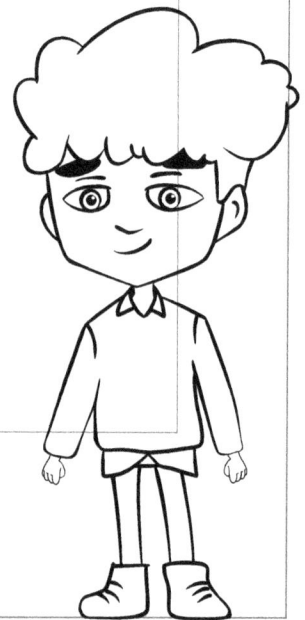

Date: _____

I can brush my teeth	I use a toothbrush
The dentist checks my teeth	My teeth are happy!

write a lil story about going to the dentist:

_____

_____

_____

Draw a picture of a happy tooth!

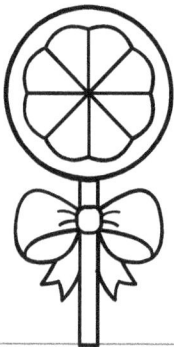

Draw a picture of dental floss:

Draw a picture of the dental office:

Draw a picture of the dental hygienist:

Date: _____

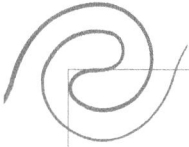

I will Floss my
teeth
everyday

Did I eat
alot of
sugar today?

How do
my teeth
feel today?

I will use
mouthwash
everyday

Write a lil story about your teeth:

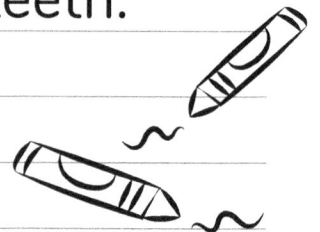

_____

_____

_____

_____

Date:

My Next Dental Cleaning Will Be:

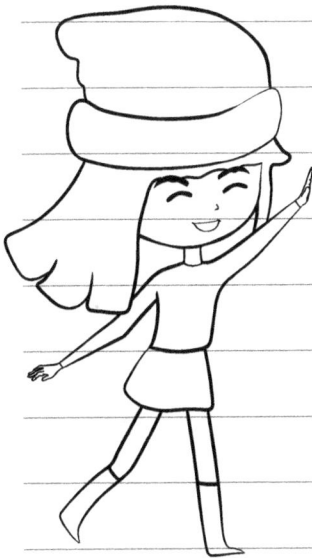

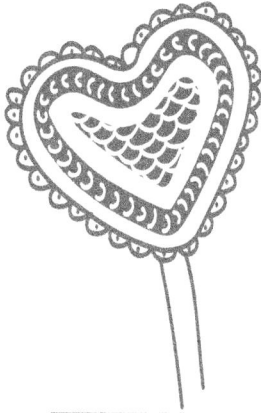

Write a note of thanks to the tooth fairy:

My tooth came out on this date

Write the amount the tooth fairy left under your pillow

Practice Writing:

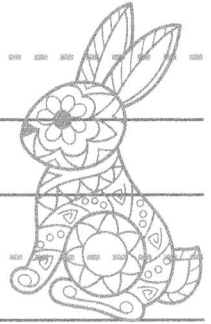

I have happy teeth

I love to brush my teeth

I love to floss my teeth

tooth

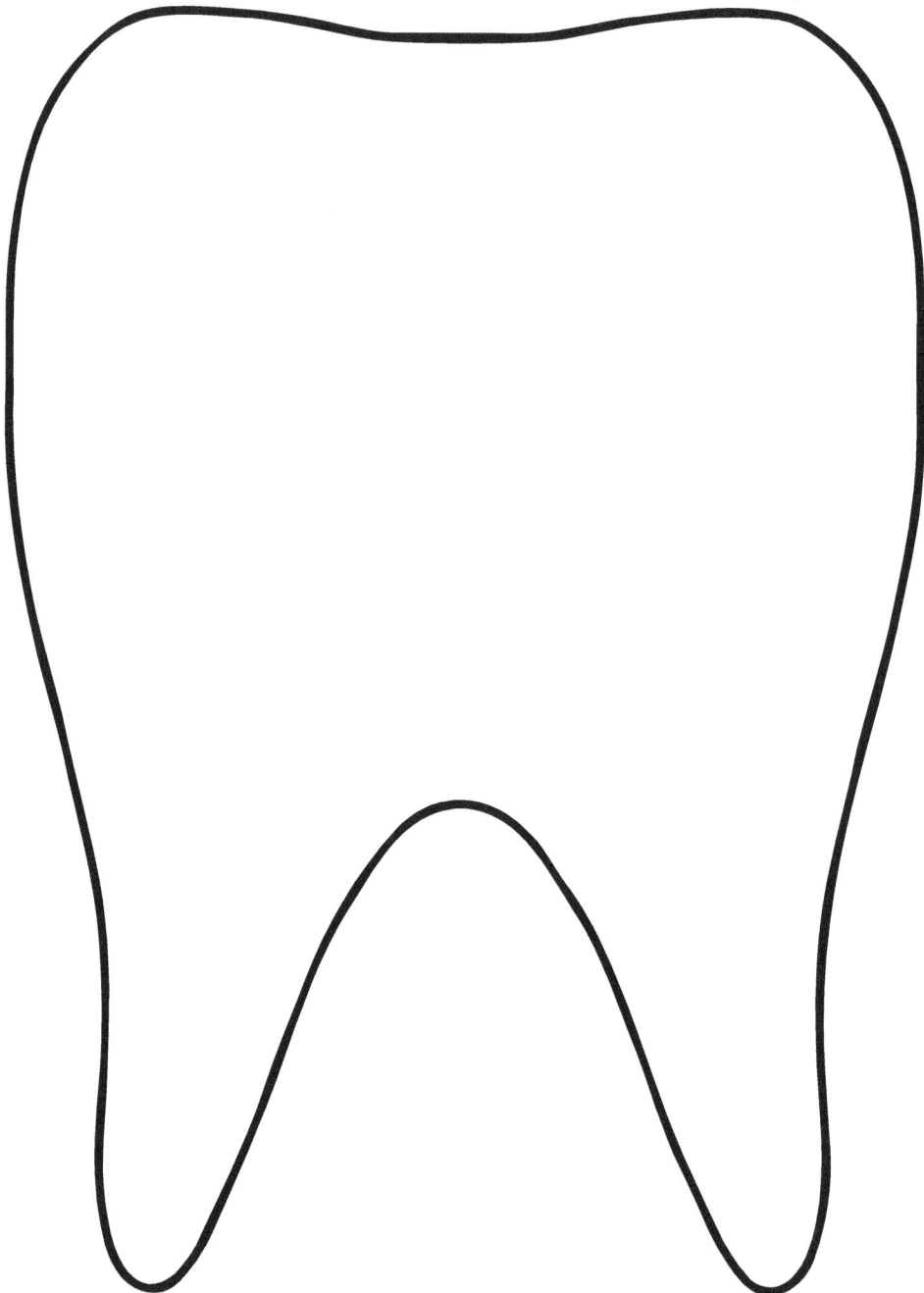

tooth x-ray

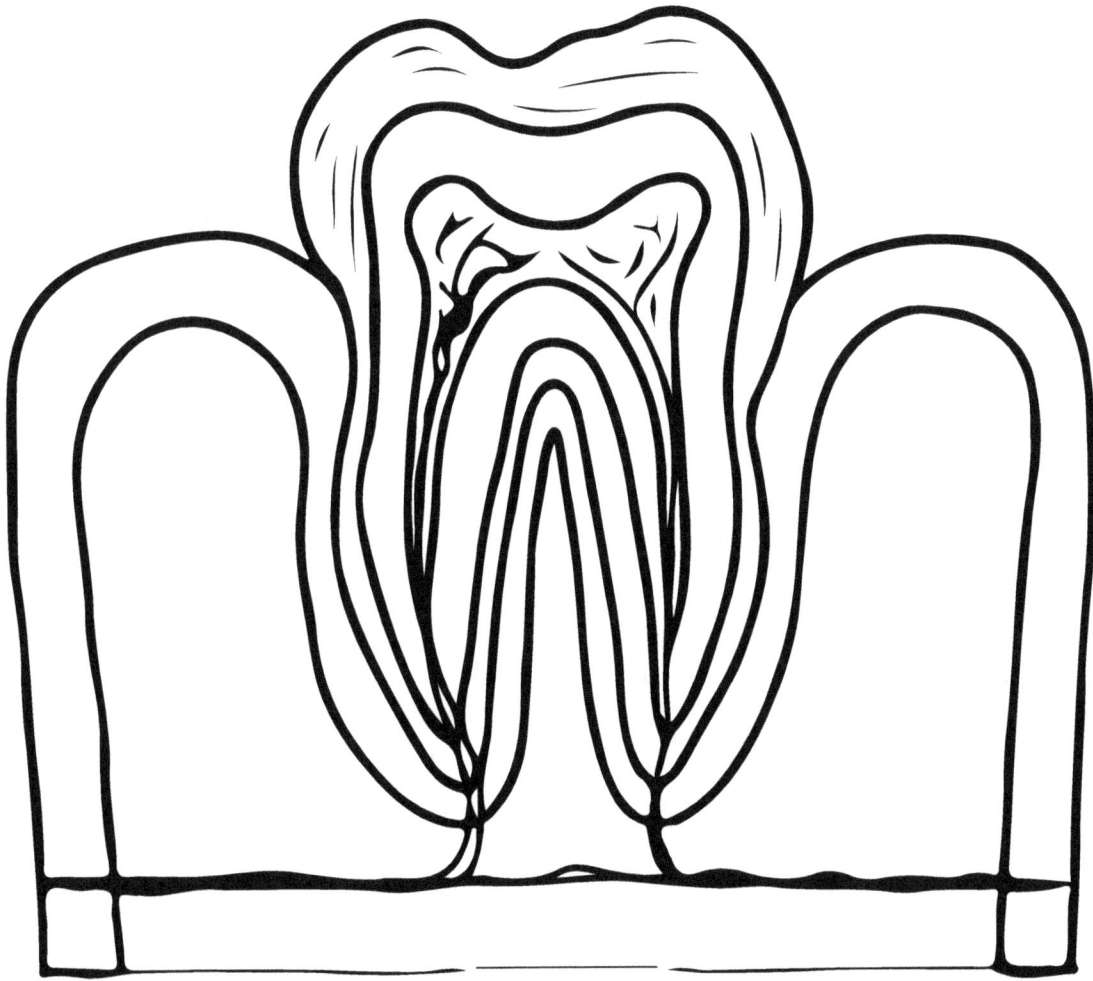

cavity

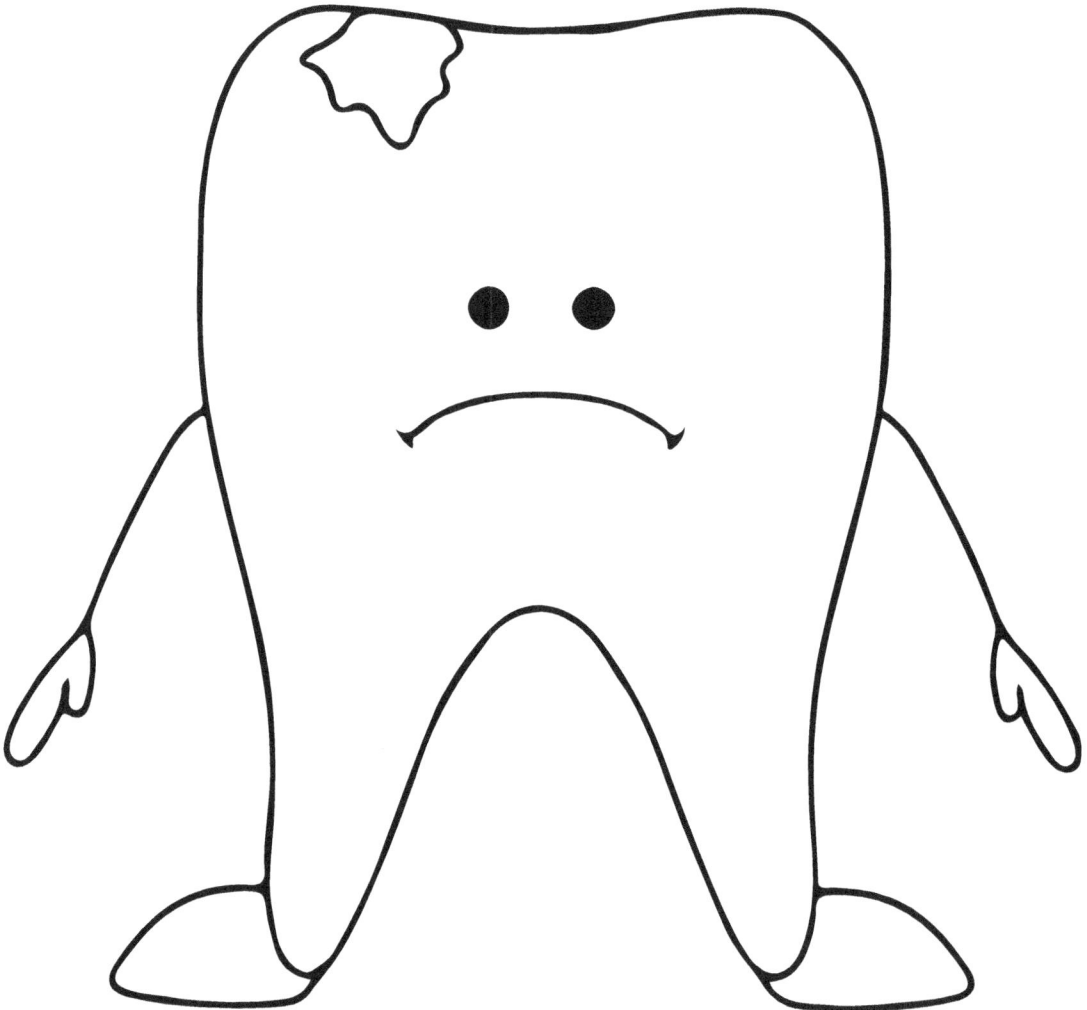

check-up

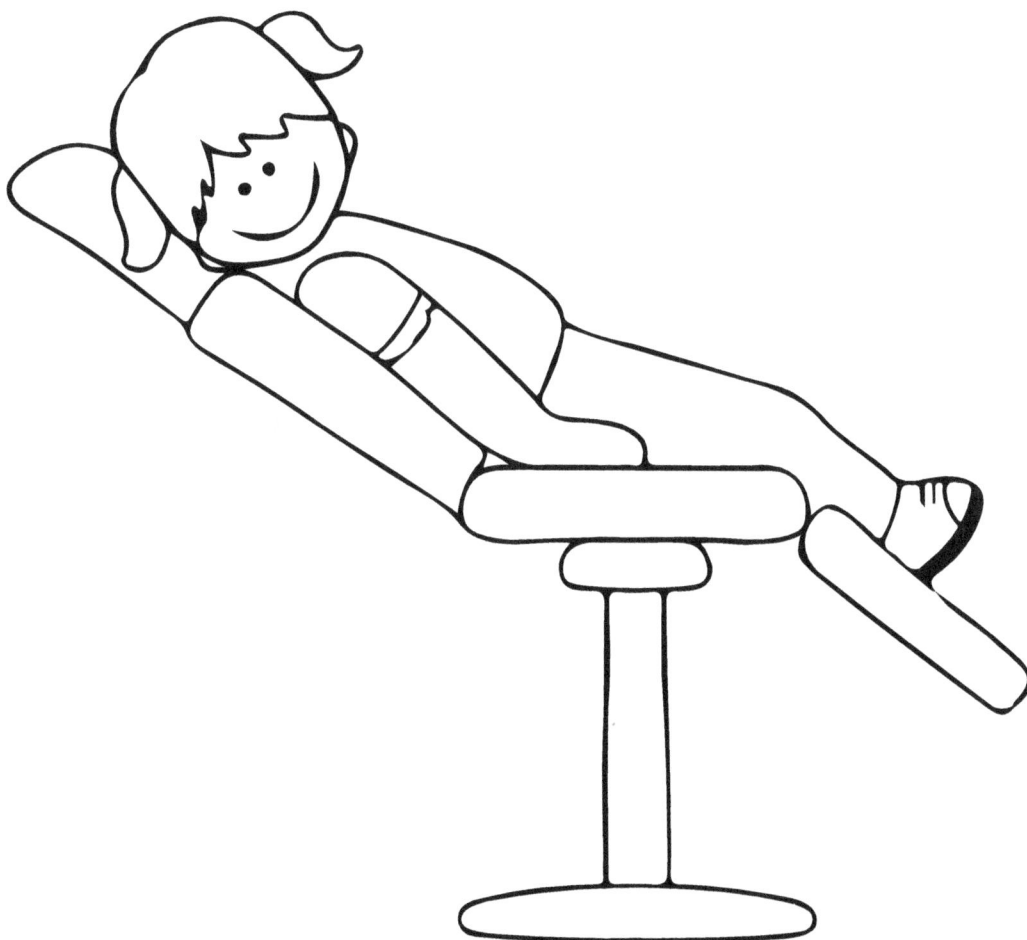

Tooth Fairy

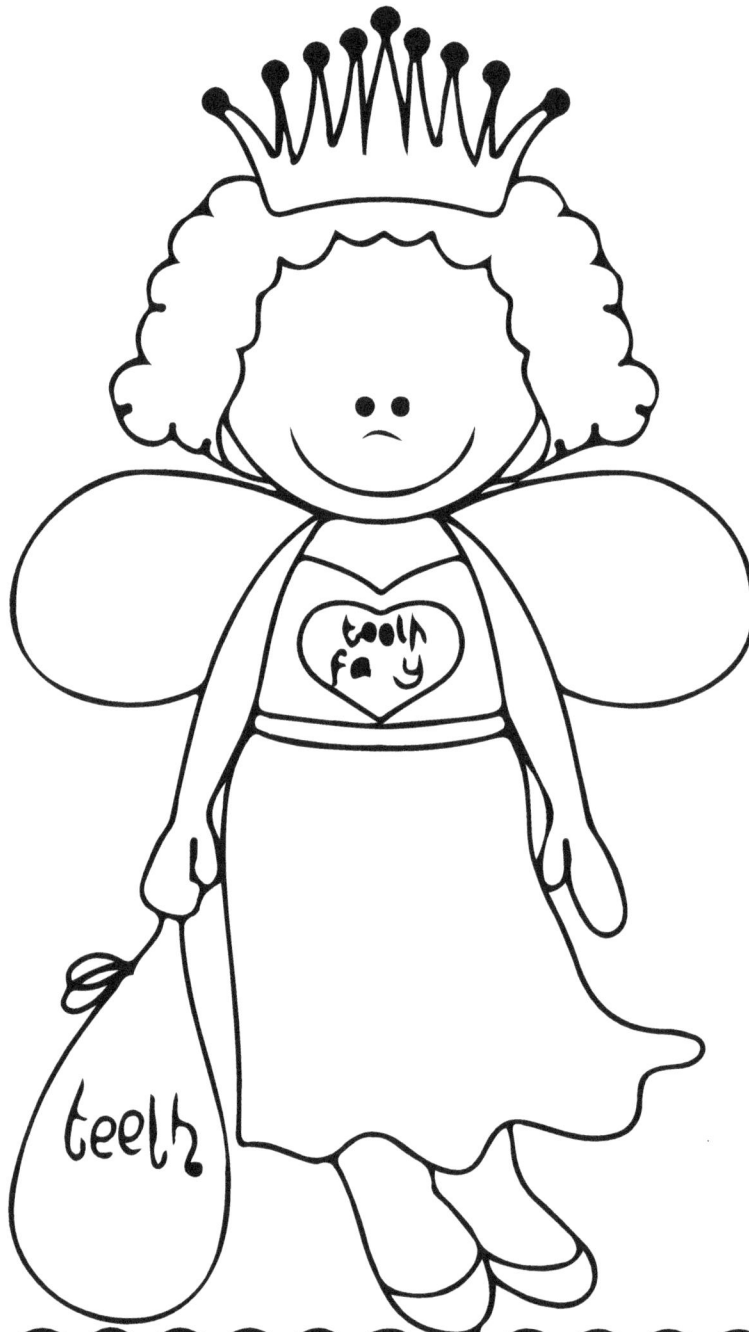

dentist

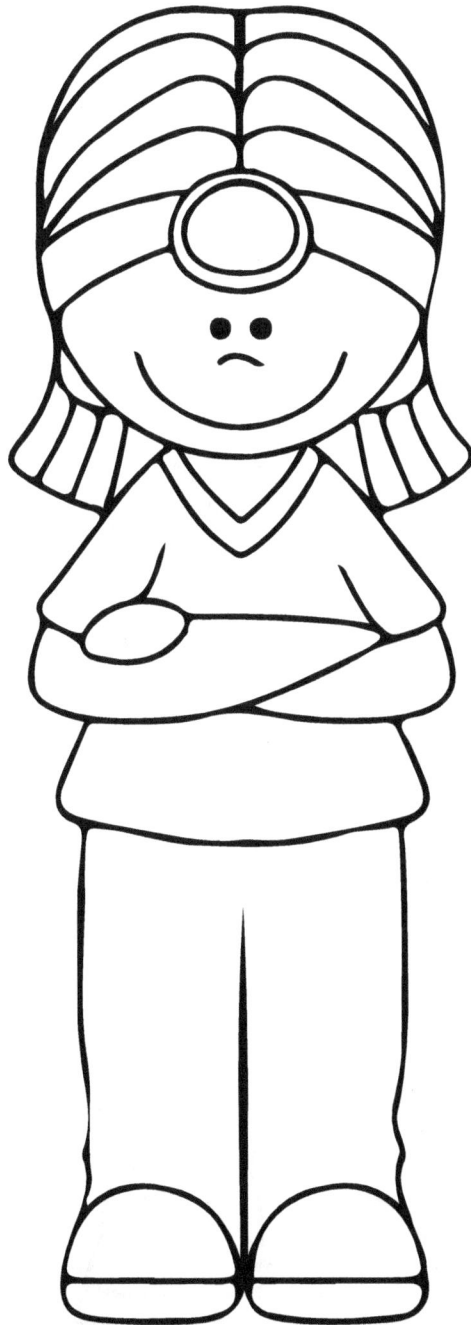

dentist

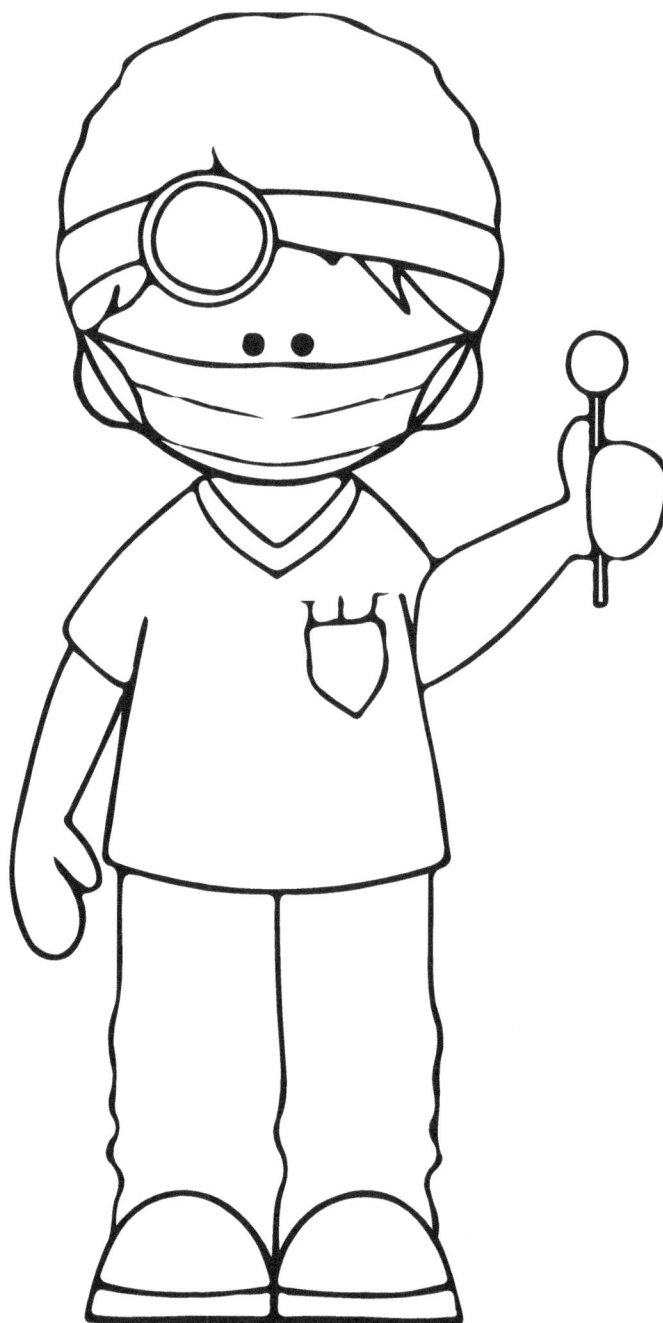

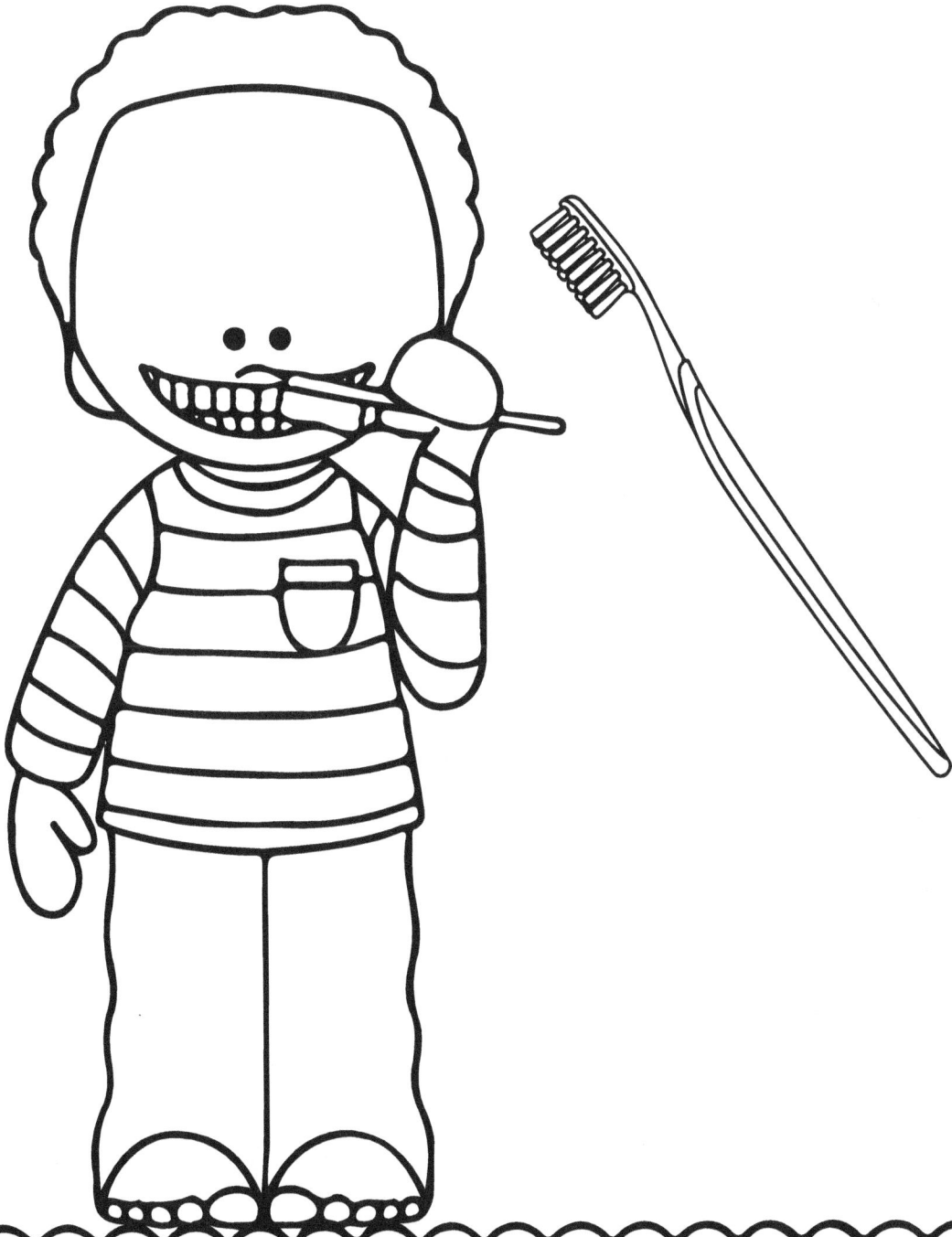

brush

brush

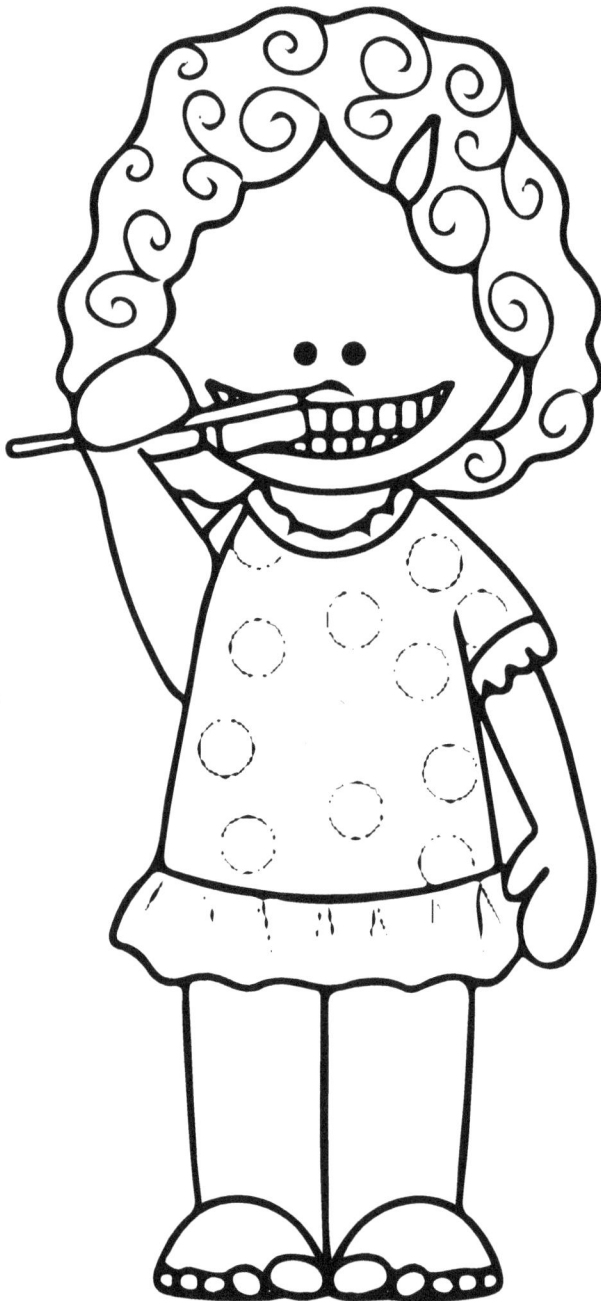
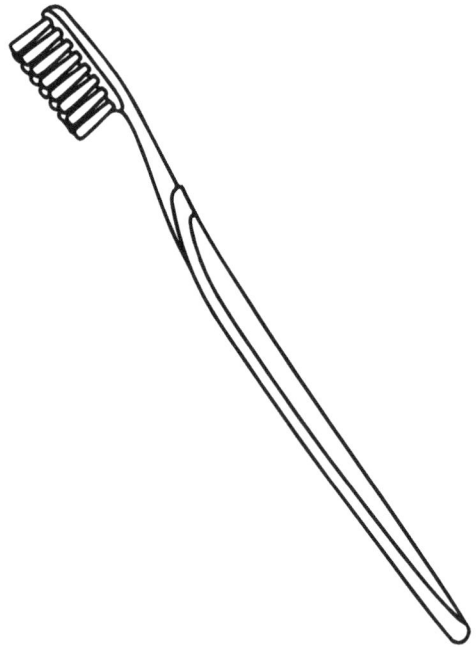

floss

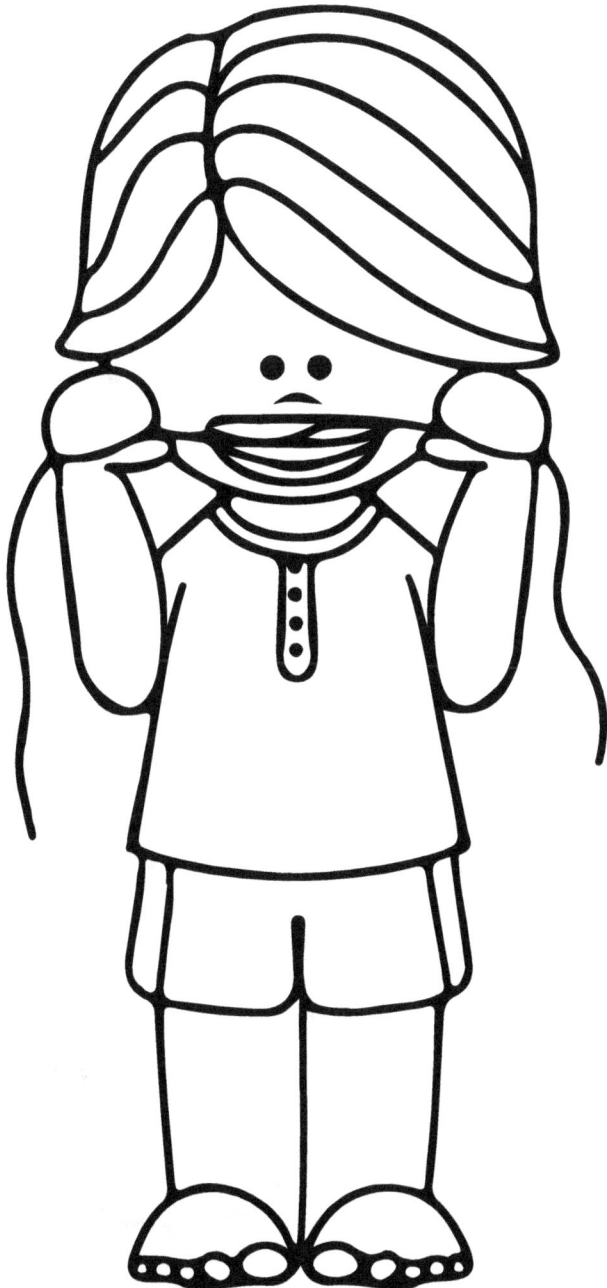

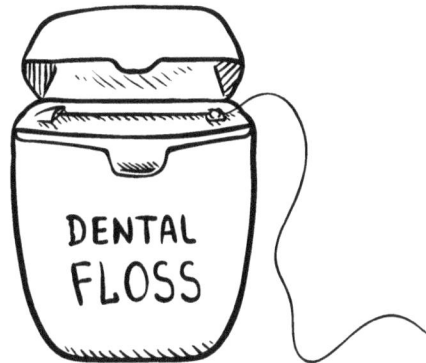

DENTAL FLOSS

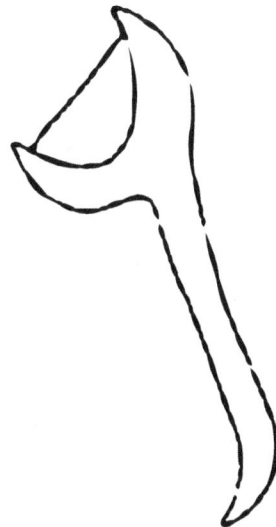

Color. Match.

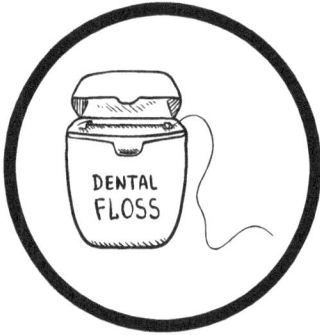

tooth

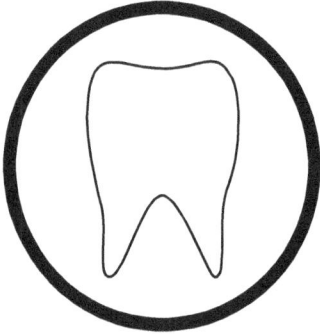

floss

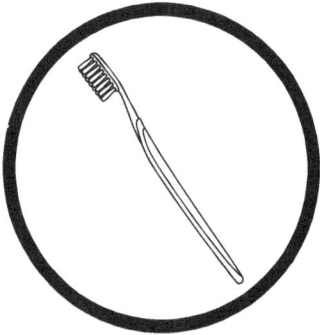

dentist

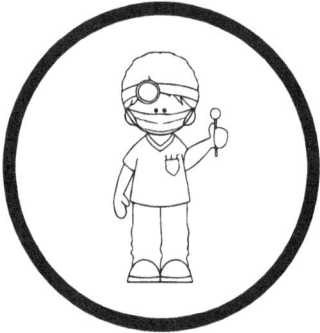

toothbrush

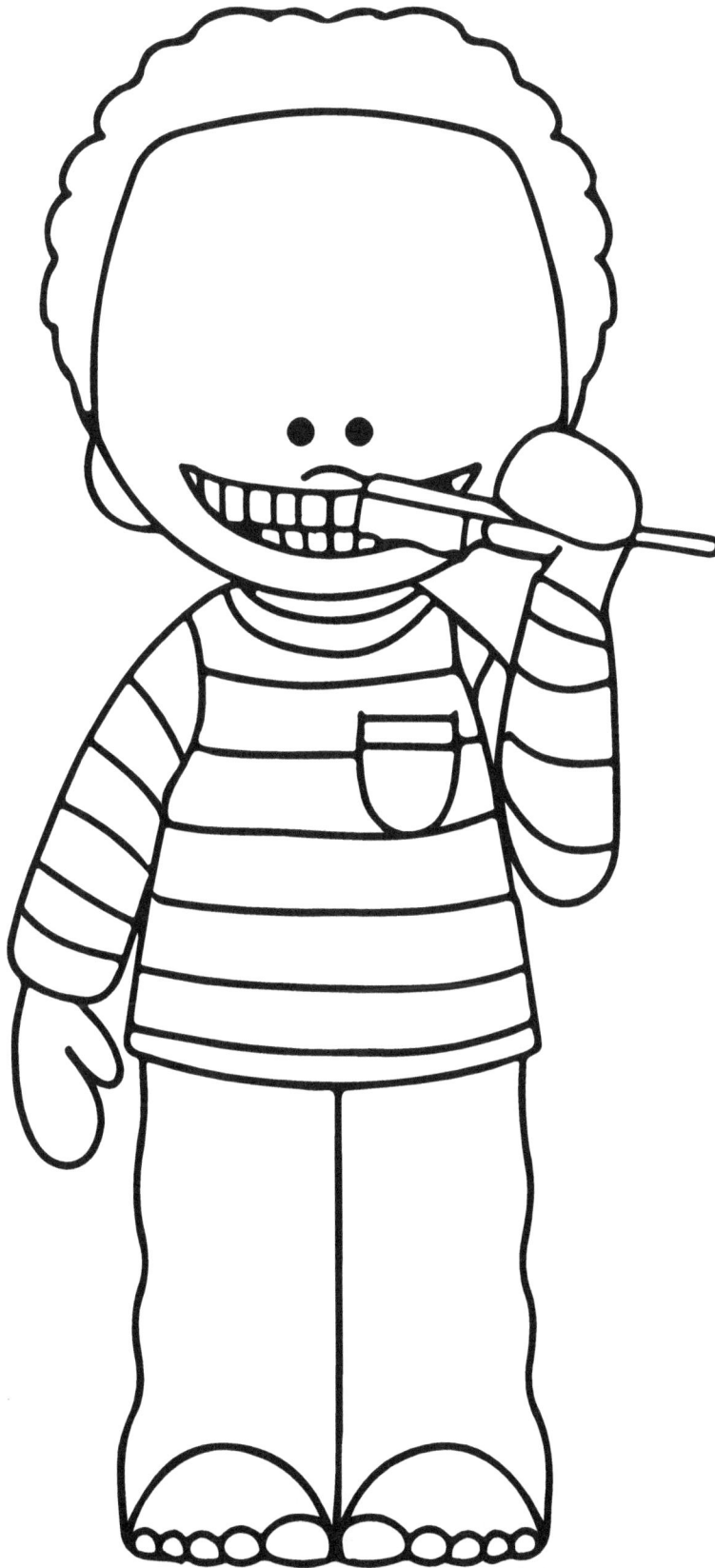

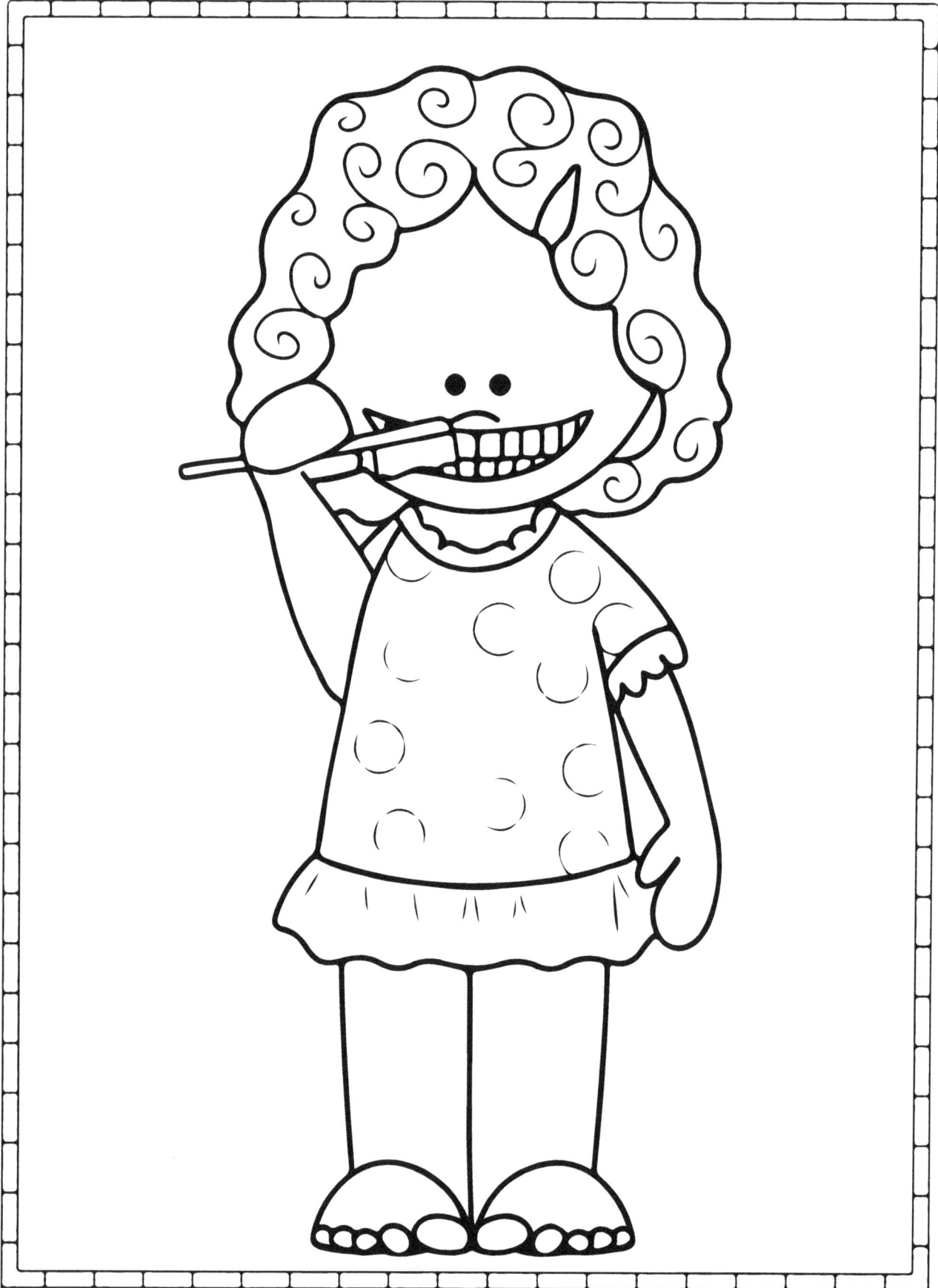

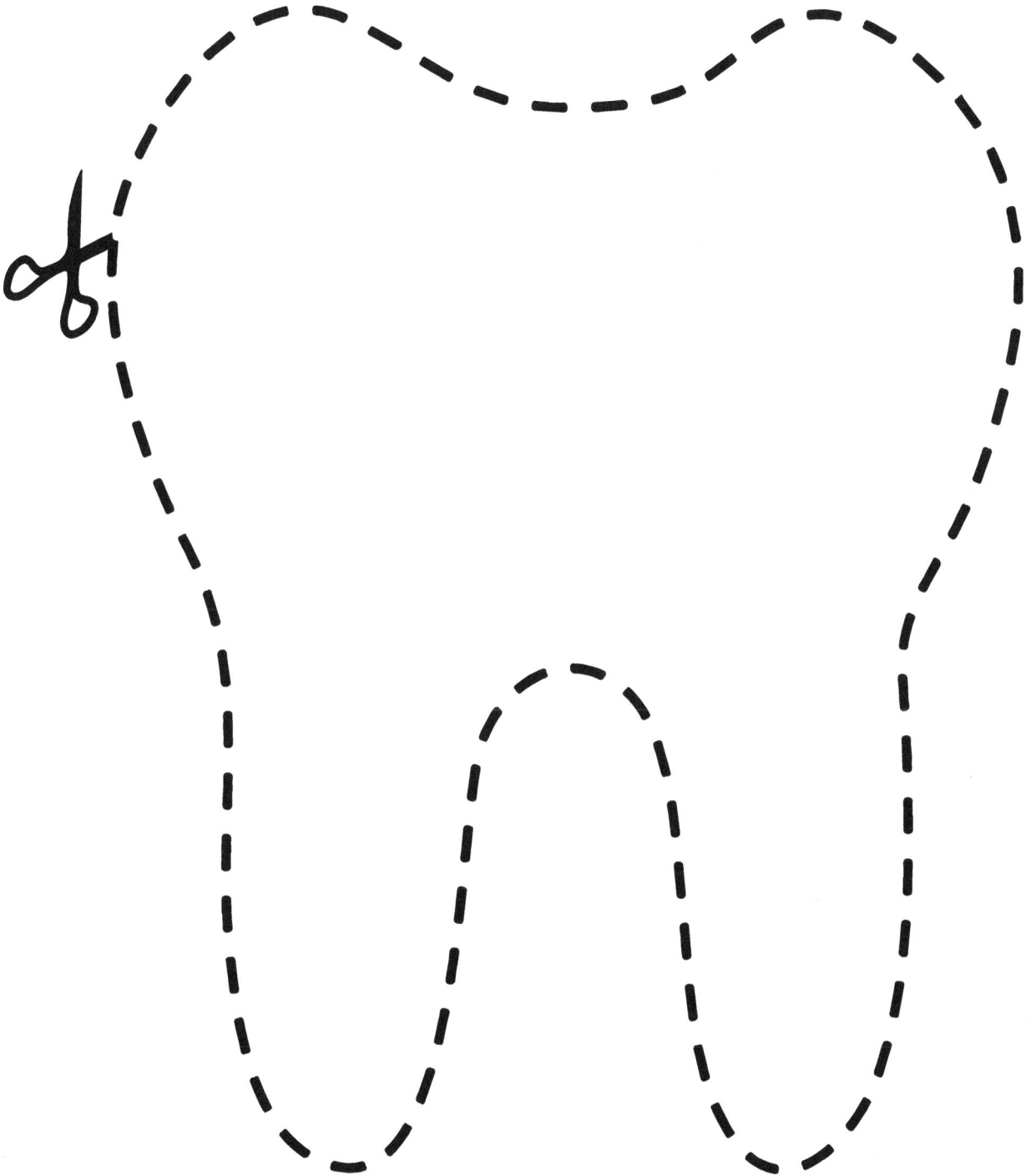

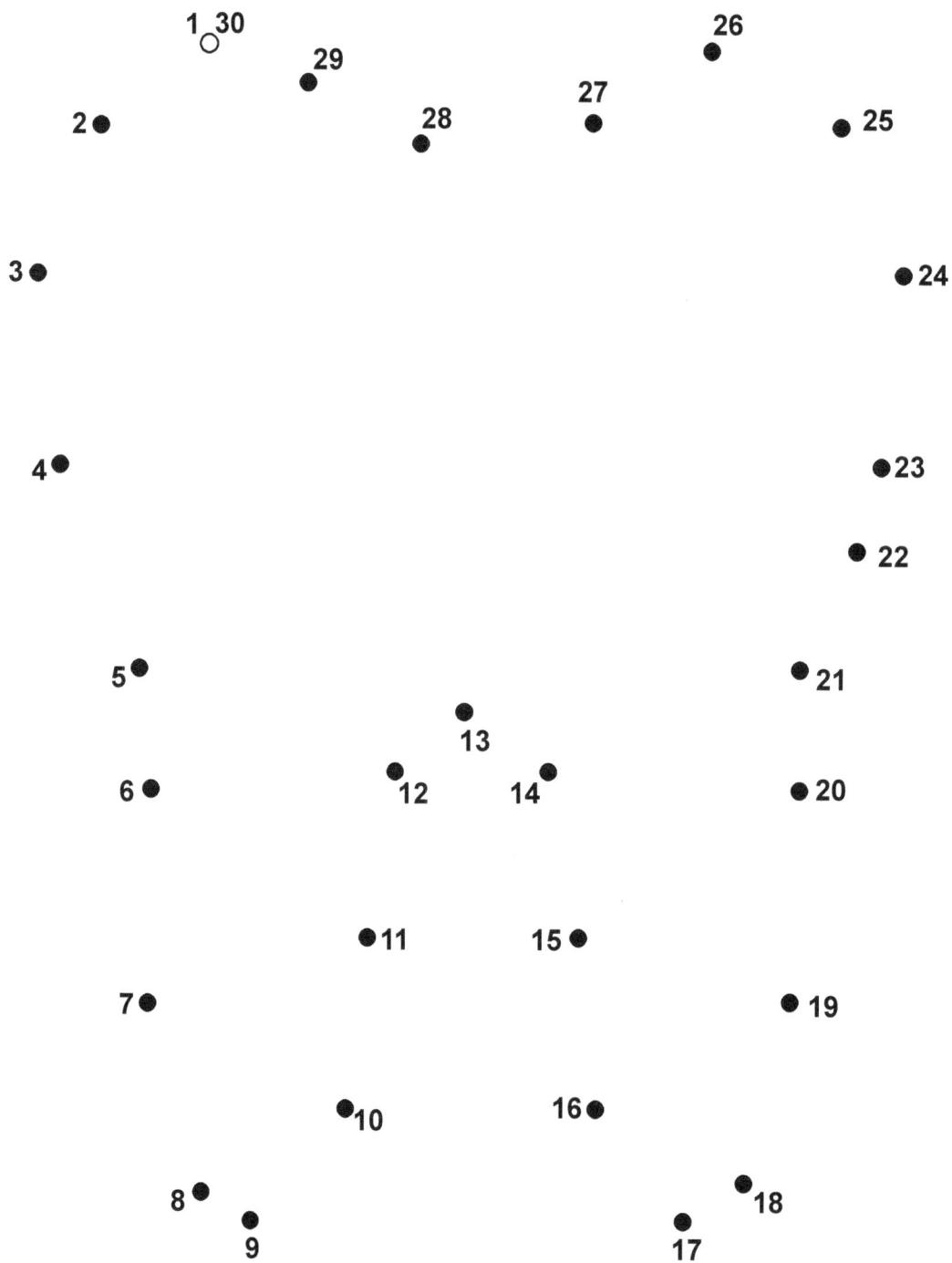

1 30

29

26

2

27

28

25

3

24

4

23

22

5

13

21

6

12

14

20

11

15

7

19

10

16

8

18

9

17

Draw a picture of a tooth:

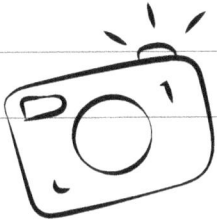

Draw a picture of your dentist

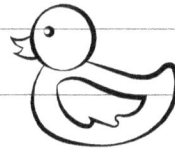

Draw a picture of your toothbrush:

Draw a picture of the tooth fairy:

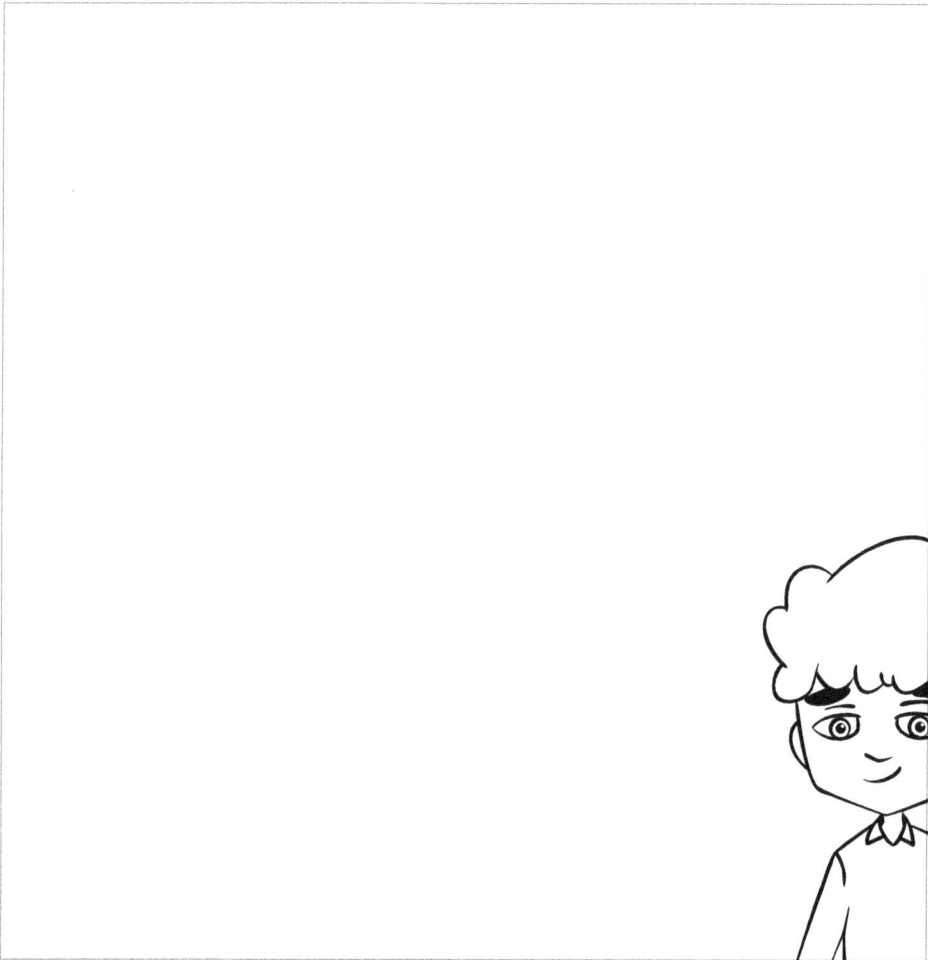

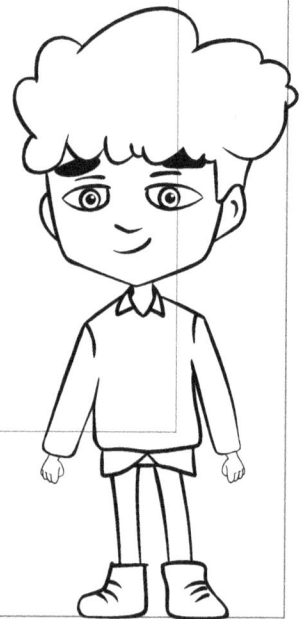

Date: _____

I can brush my teeth	I use a toothbrush
The dentist checks my teeth	My teeth are happy!

write a lil story about going to the dentist:

_____

_____

_____

Draw a picture of a happy tooth!

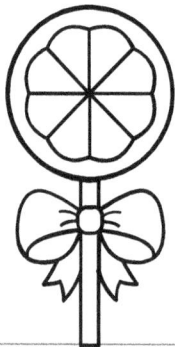

Draw a picture of dental floss:

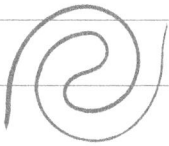

Draw a picture of the dental office:

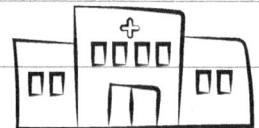

Draw a picture of the dental hygienist:

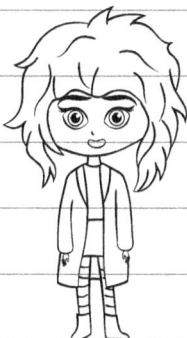

Date: _____

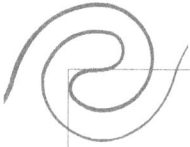

I will Floss my teeth everyday

Did I eat alot of sugar today?

How do my teeth feel today?

I will use mouthwash everyday

Write a lil story about your teeth:

_____
_____
_____
_____

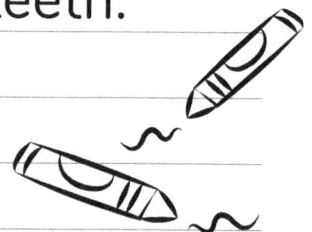

Date: _____

My Next Dental Cleaning Will Be:

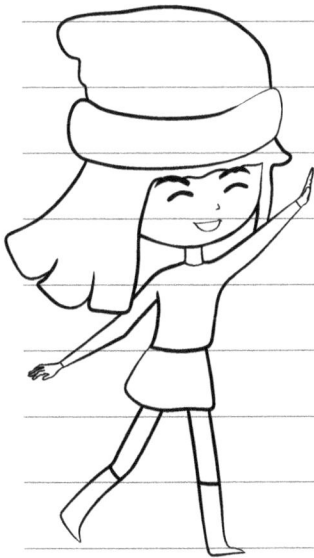

_____

_____

_____

_____

_____

_____

_____

_____

_____

_____

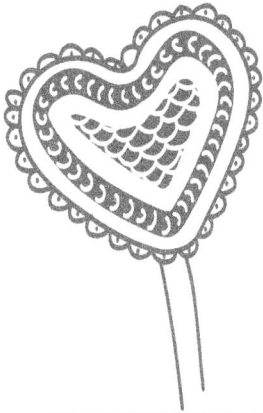

Write a note of thanks to the tooth fairy:

My tooth came out on this date

Write the amount the tooth fairy left under your pillow

Practice Writing:

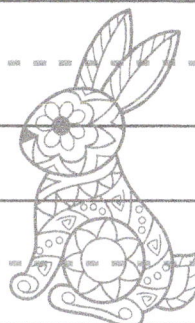

I have happy teeth

I love to brush my teeth

I love to floss my teeth

tooth

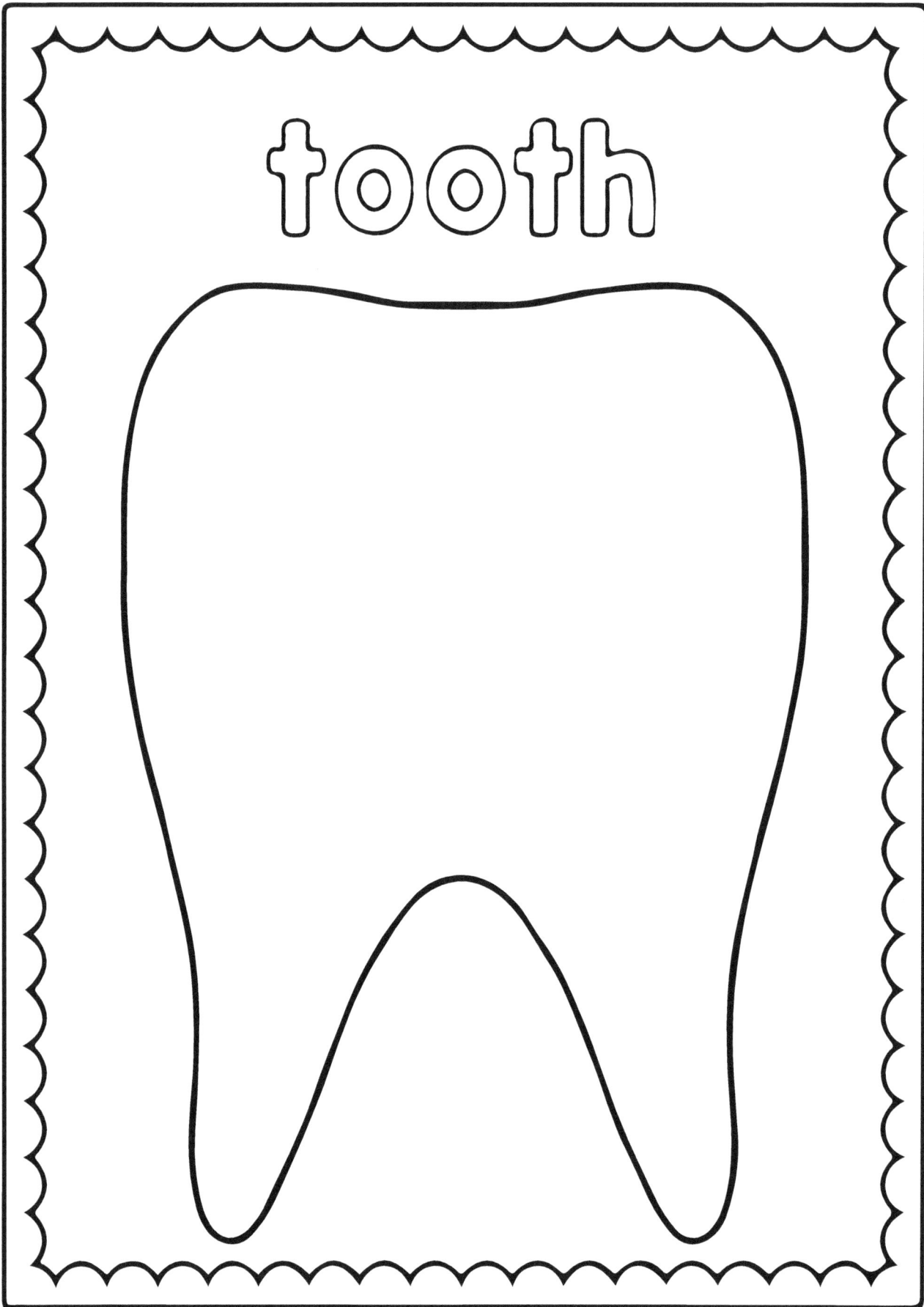

tooth x-ray

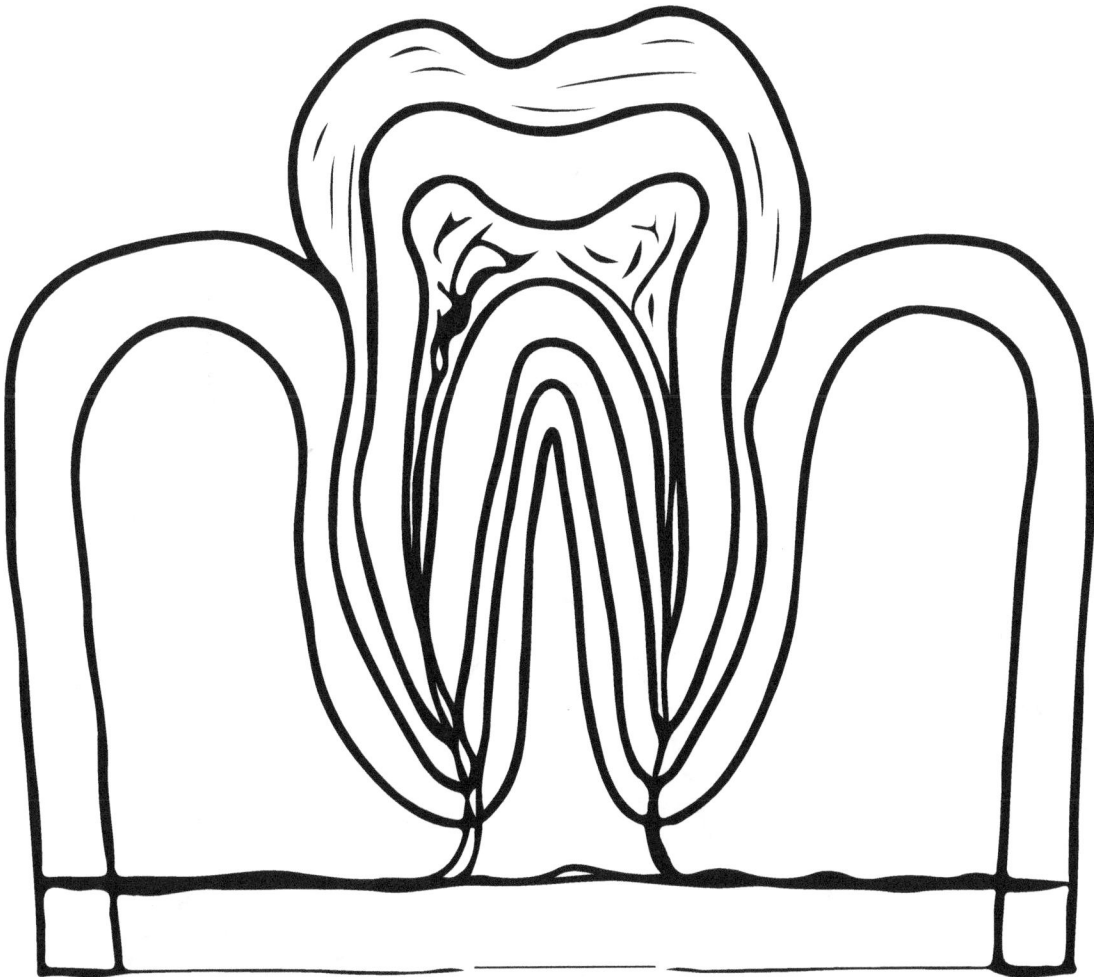

cavity

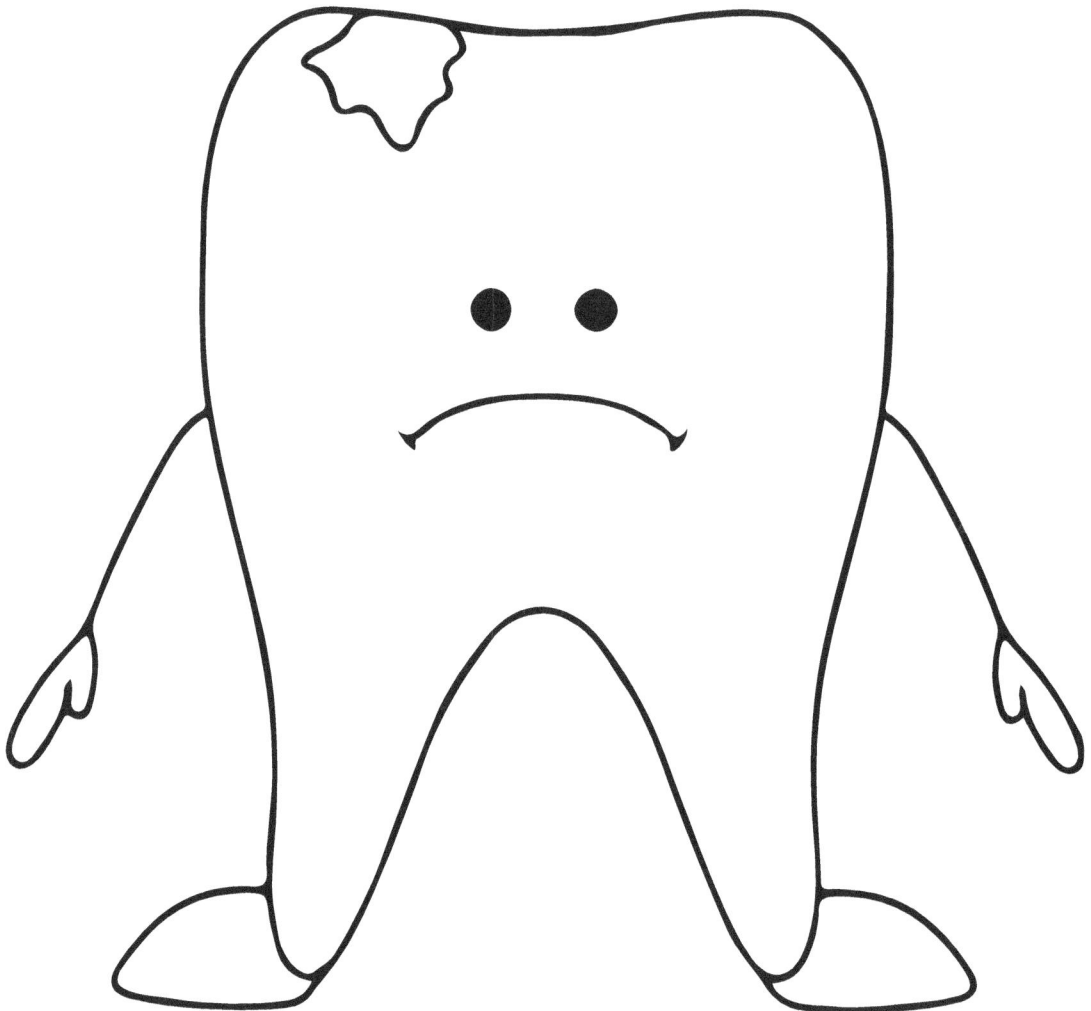

check-up

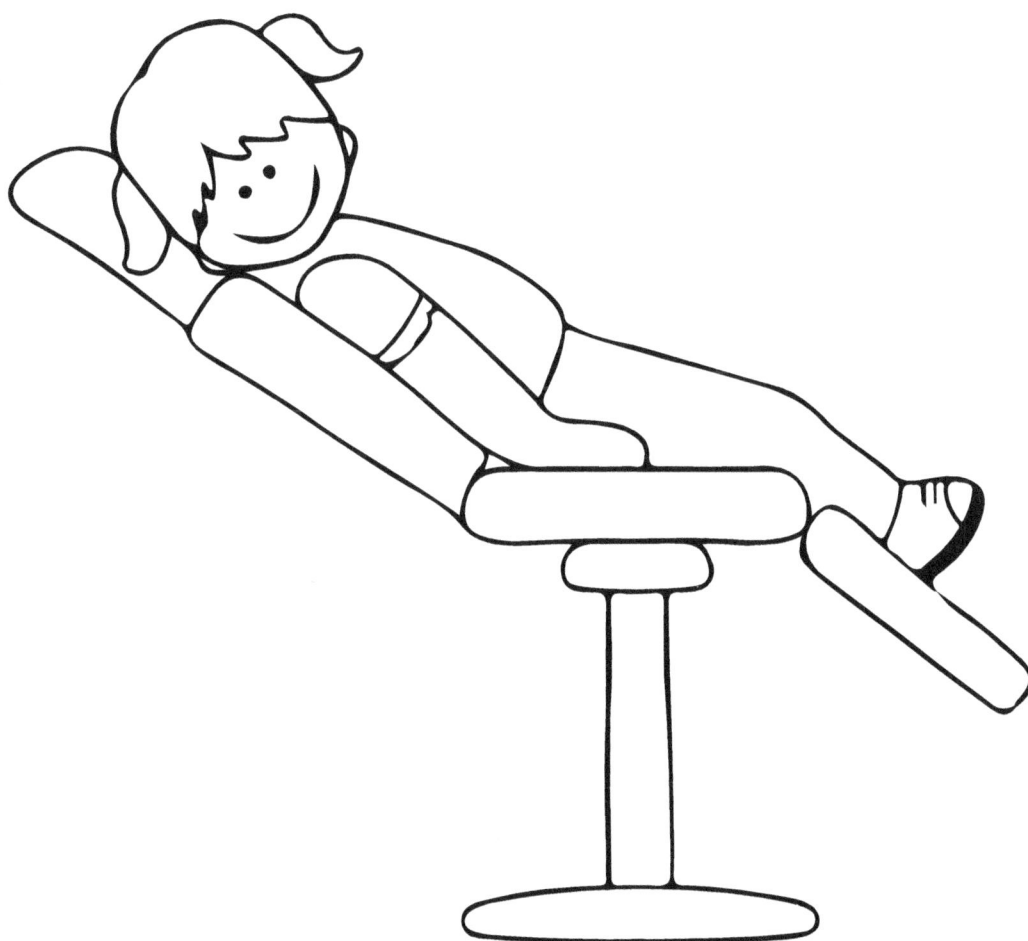

Tooth Fairy

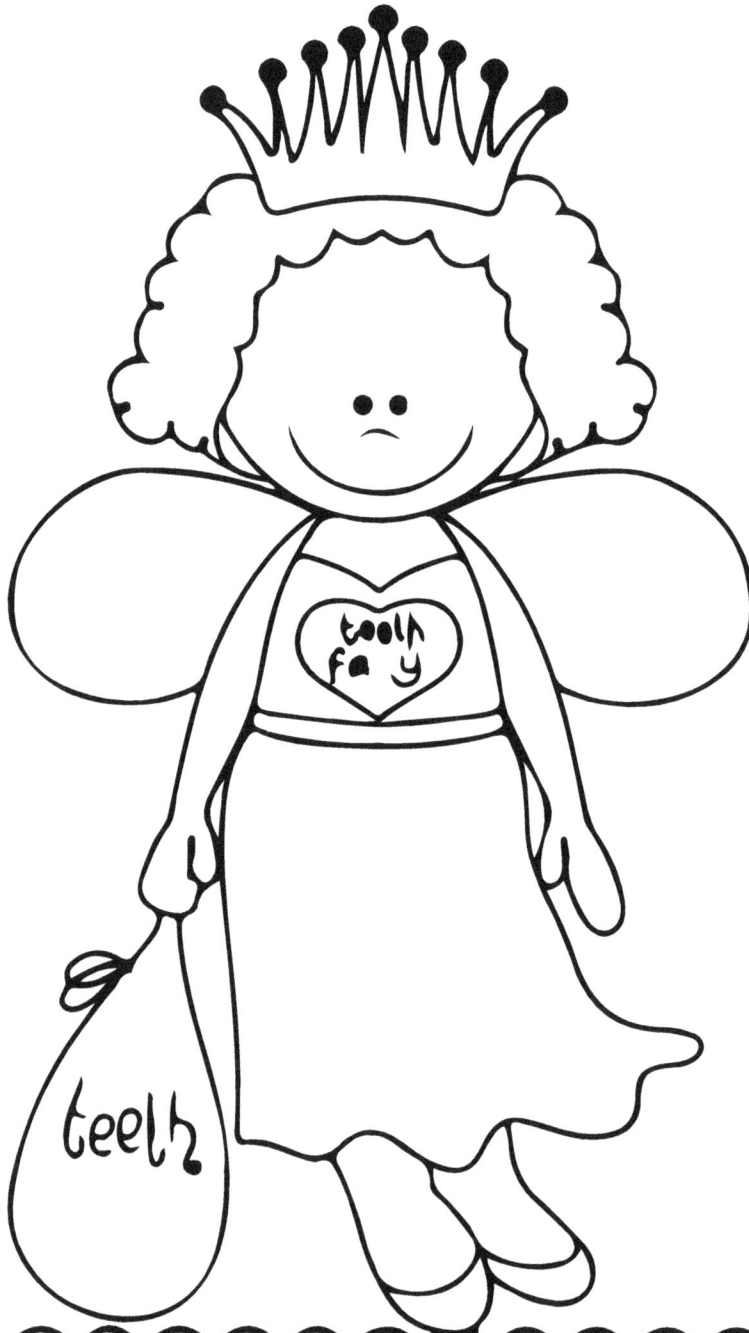

dentist

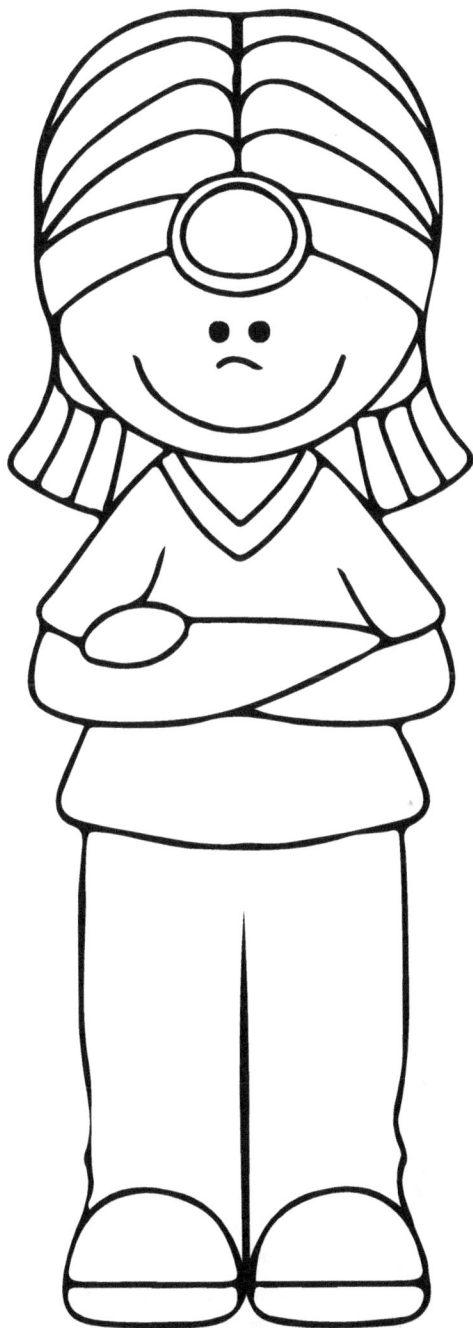

dentist

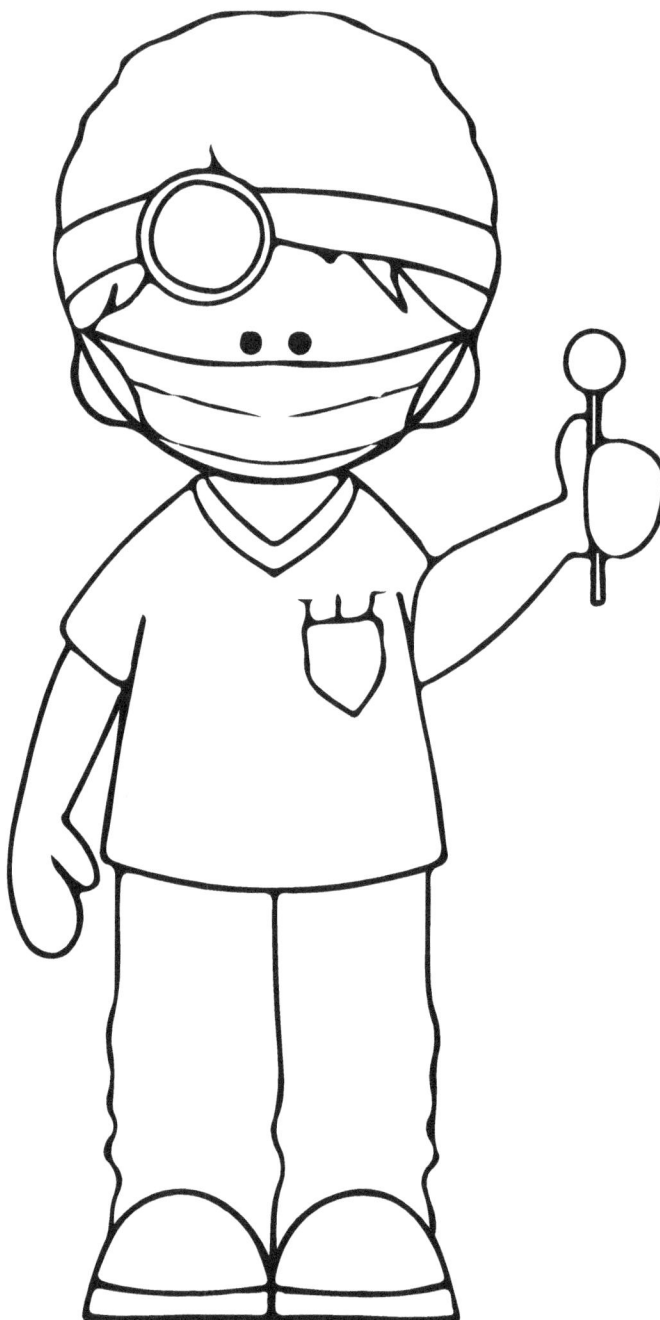

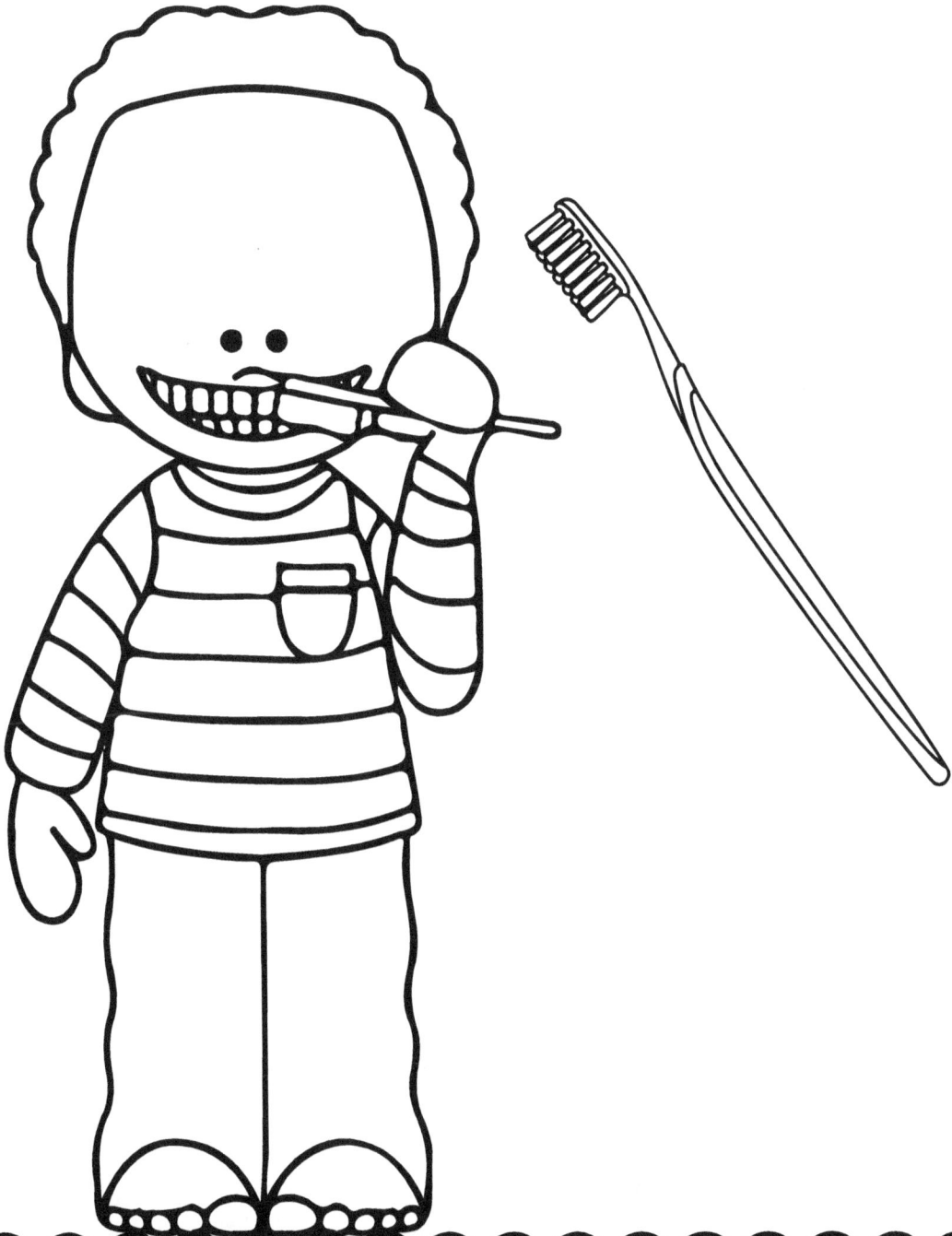

brush

brush

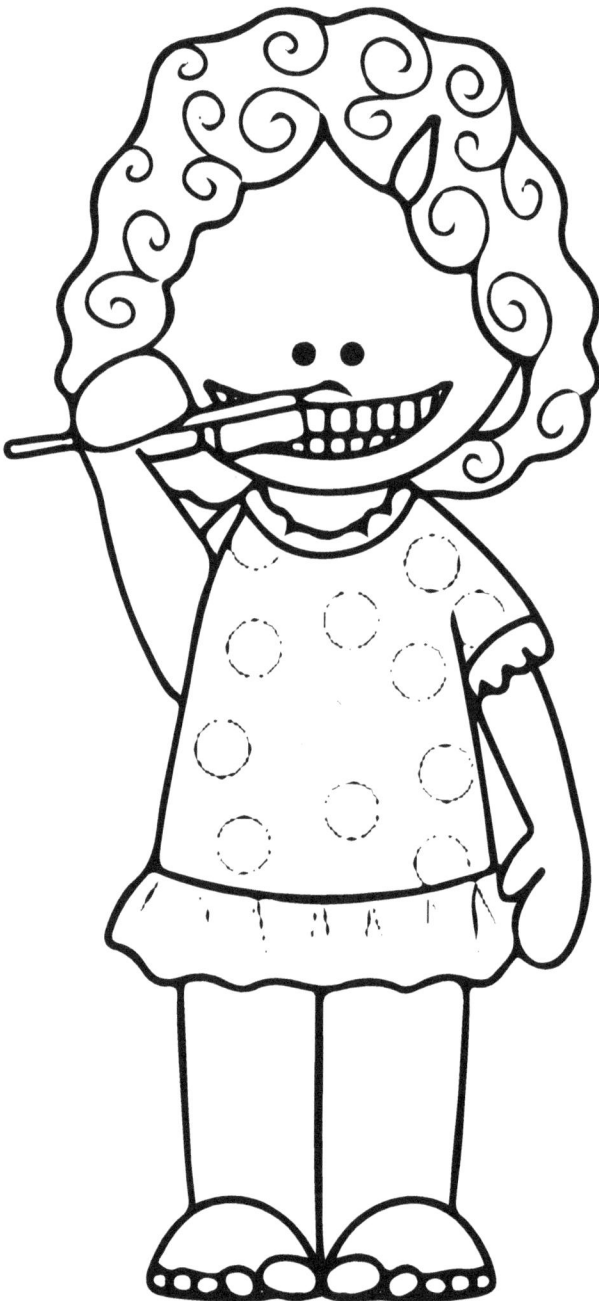
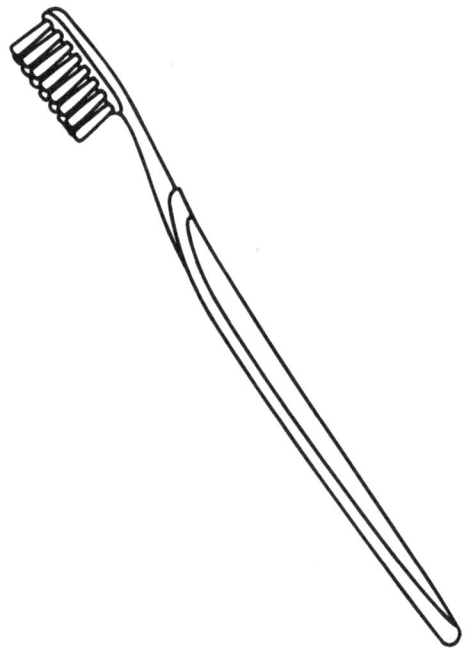

floss

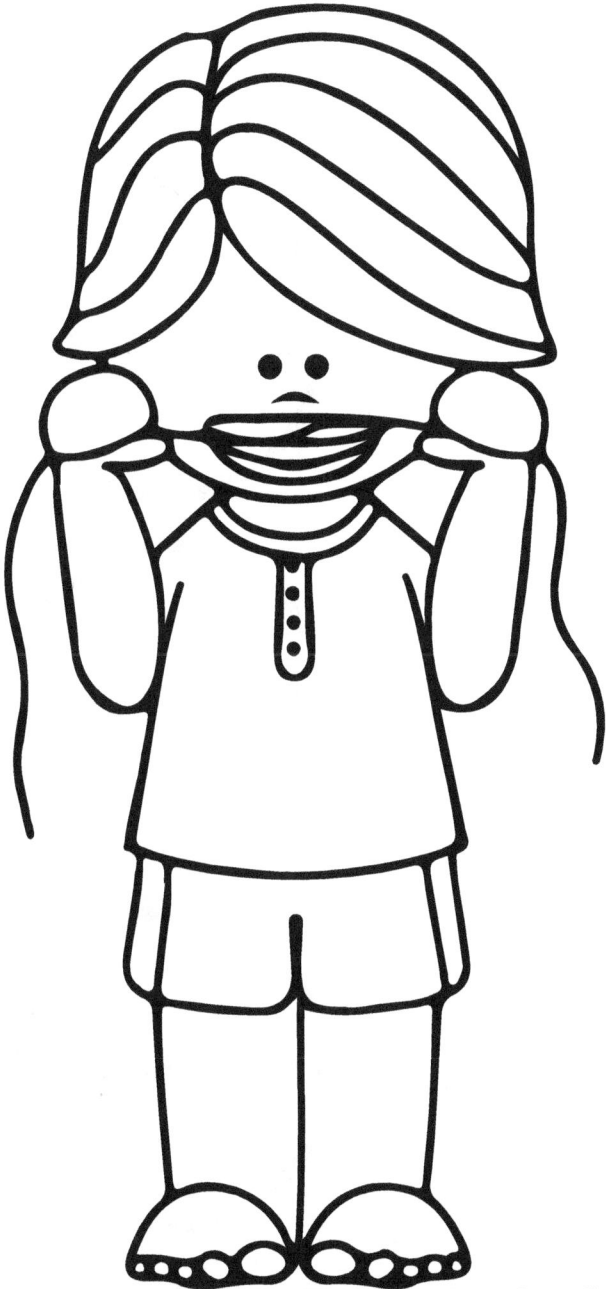
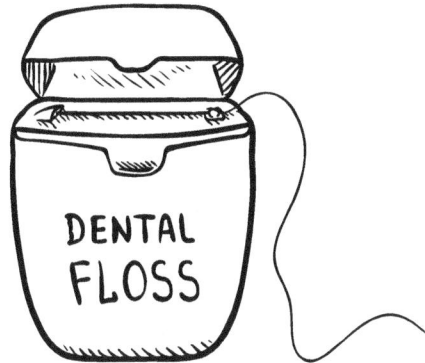

DENTAL FLOSS

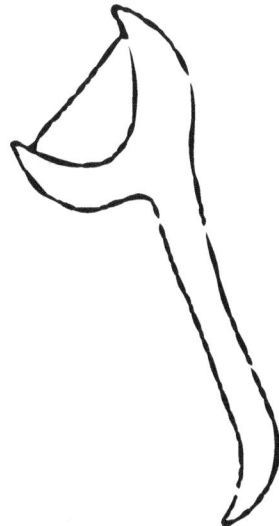

Color. Match.

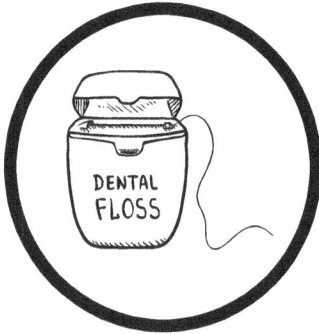

tooth

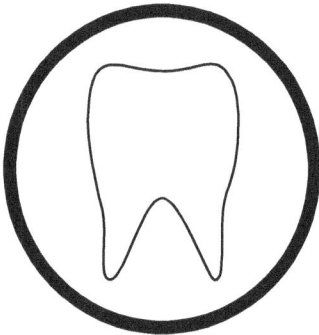

floss

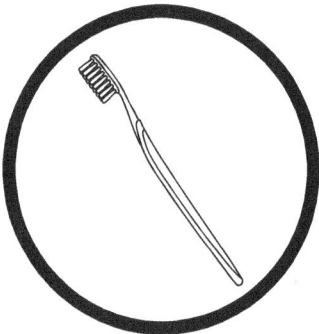

dentist

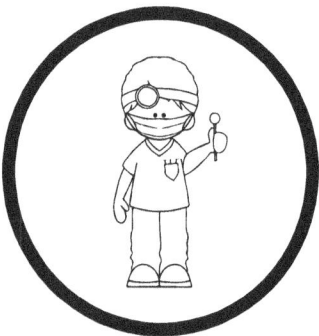

toothbrush

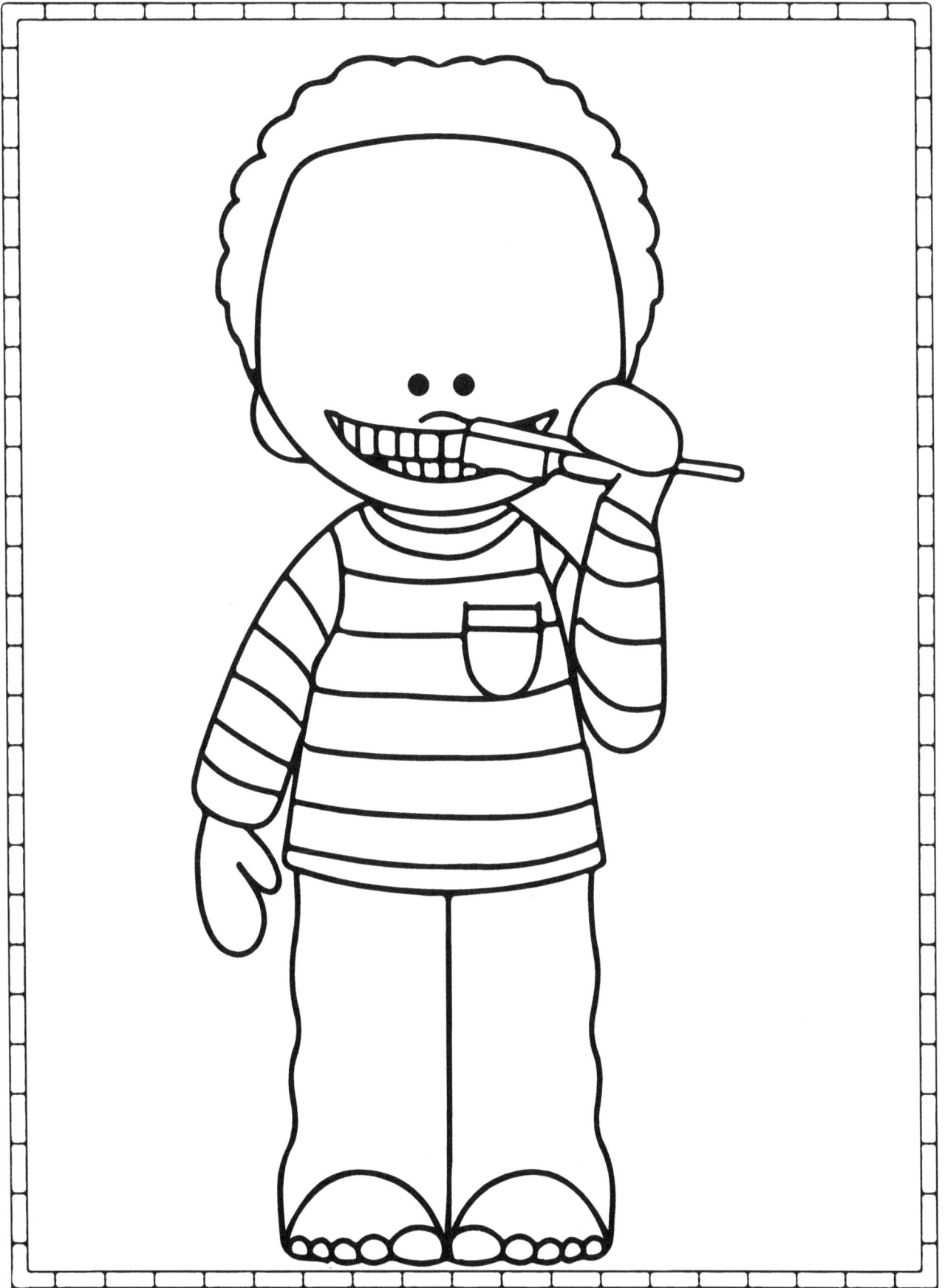

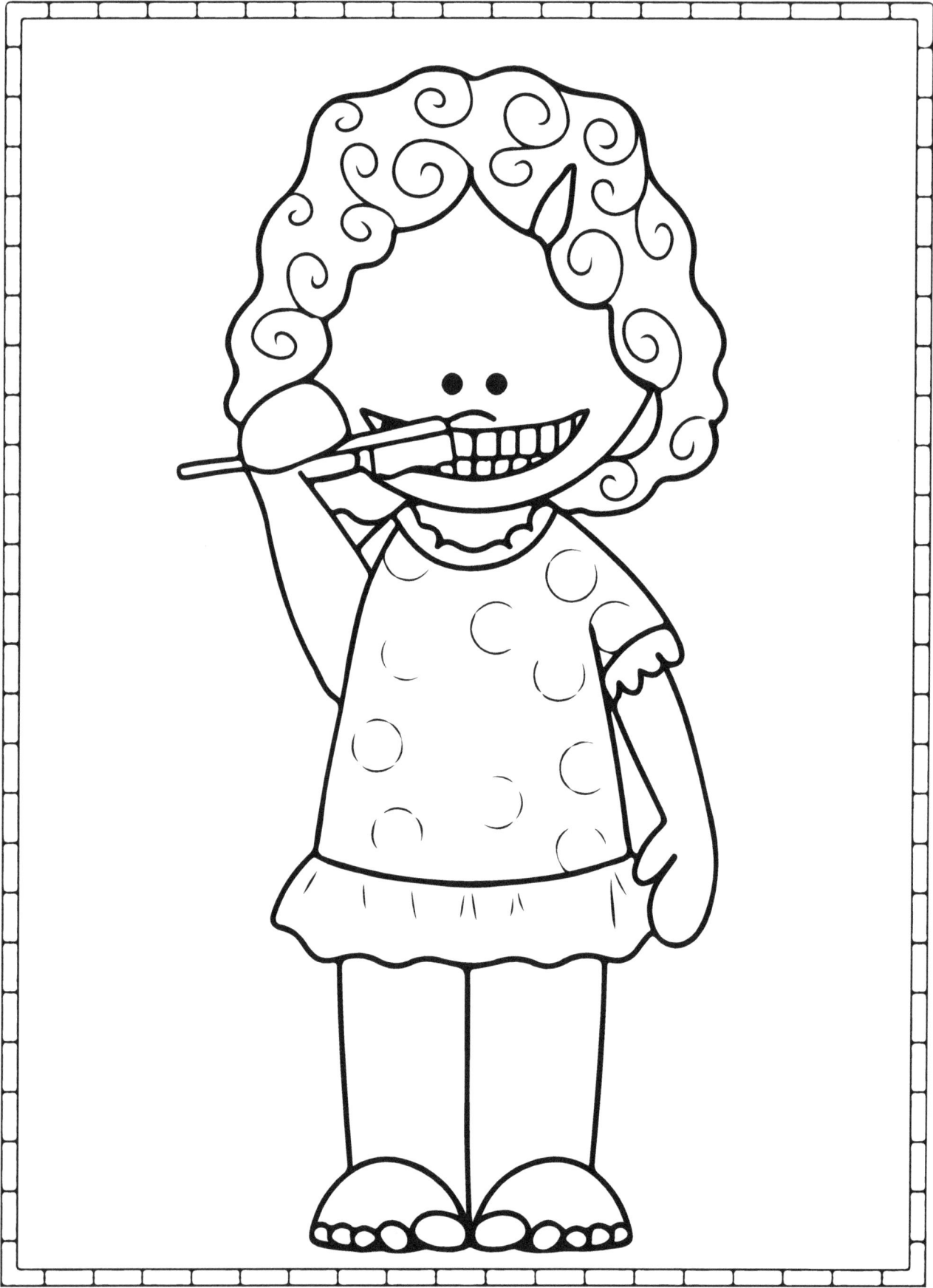

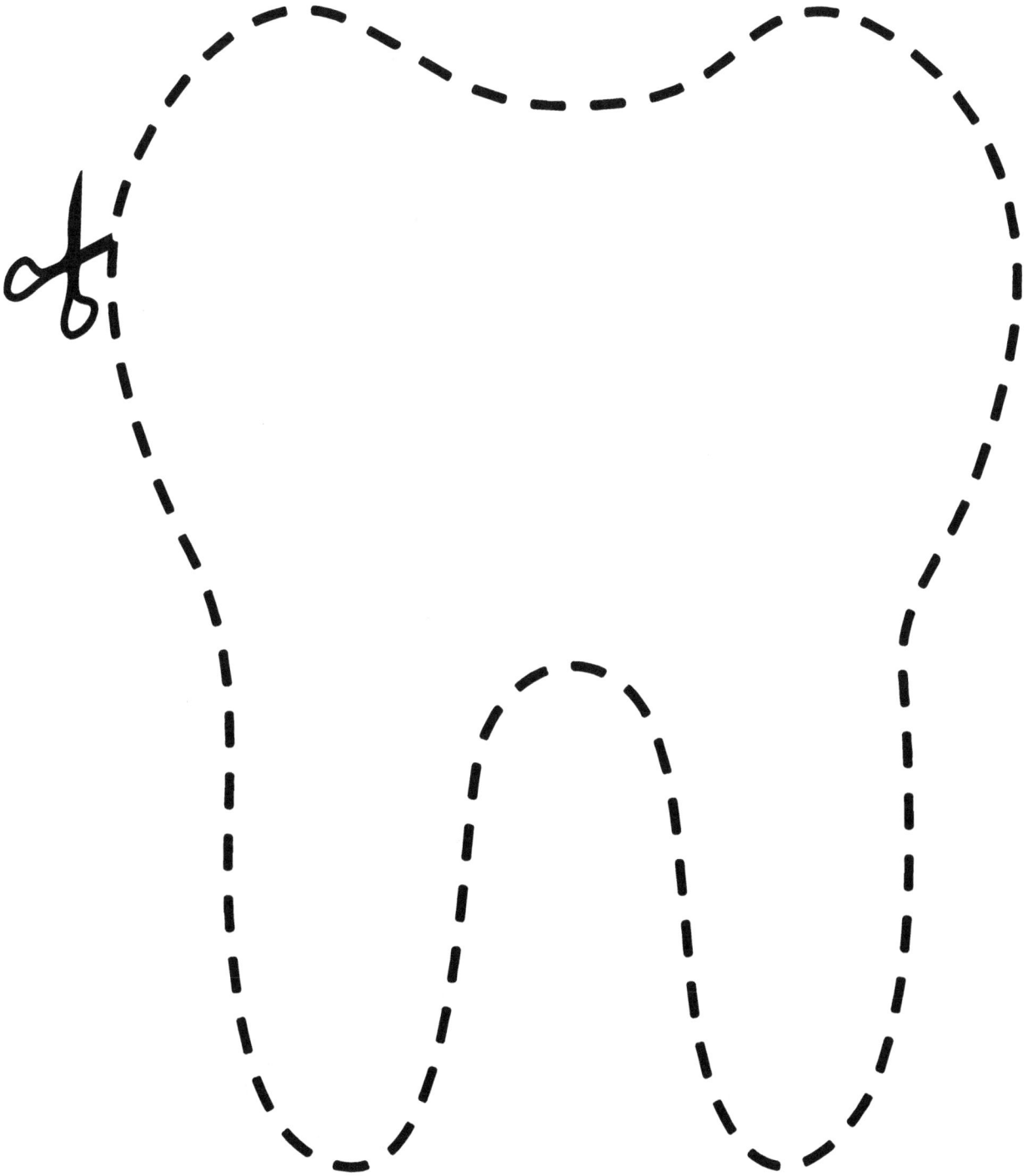

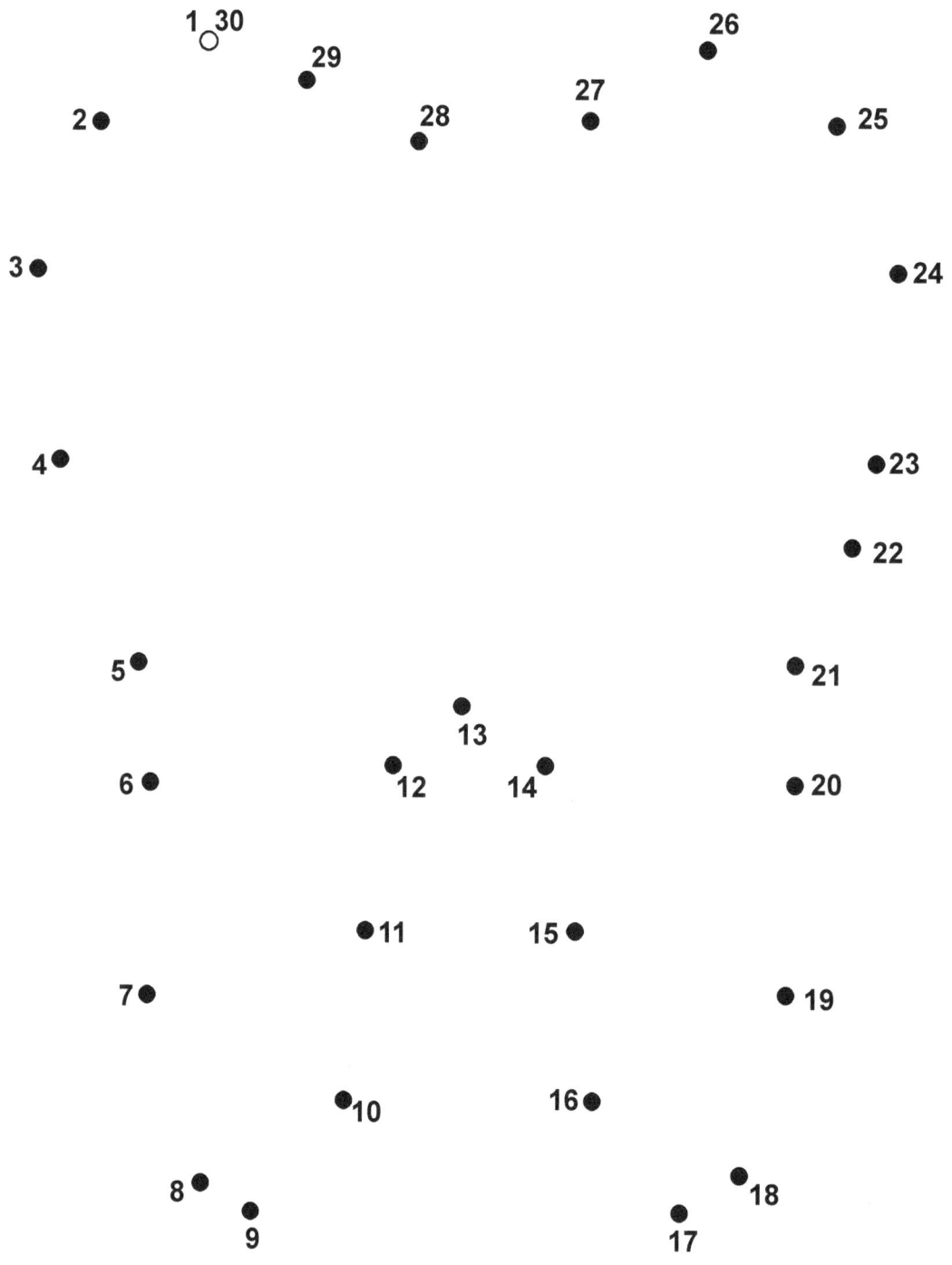

1 30
26
29
27
2 28
25
3 24
4 23
22
5 21
13
6 12 14 20
11 15
7 19
16
10
18
8 17
9

Draw a picture of a tooth:

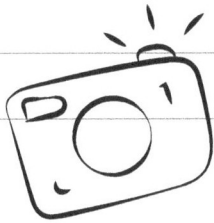

Draw a picture of your dentist

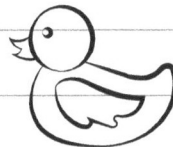

Draw a picture of your toothbrush:

Draw a picture of the tooth fairy:

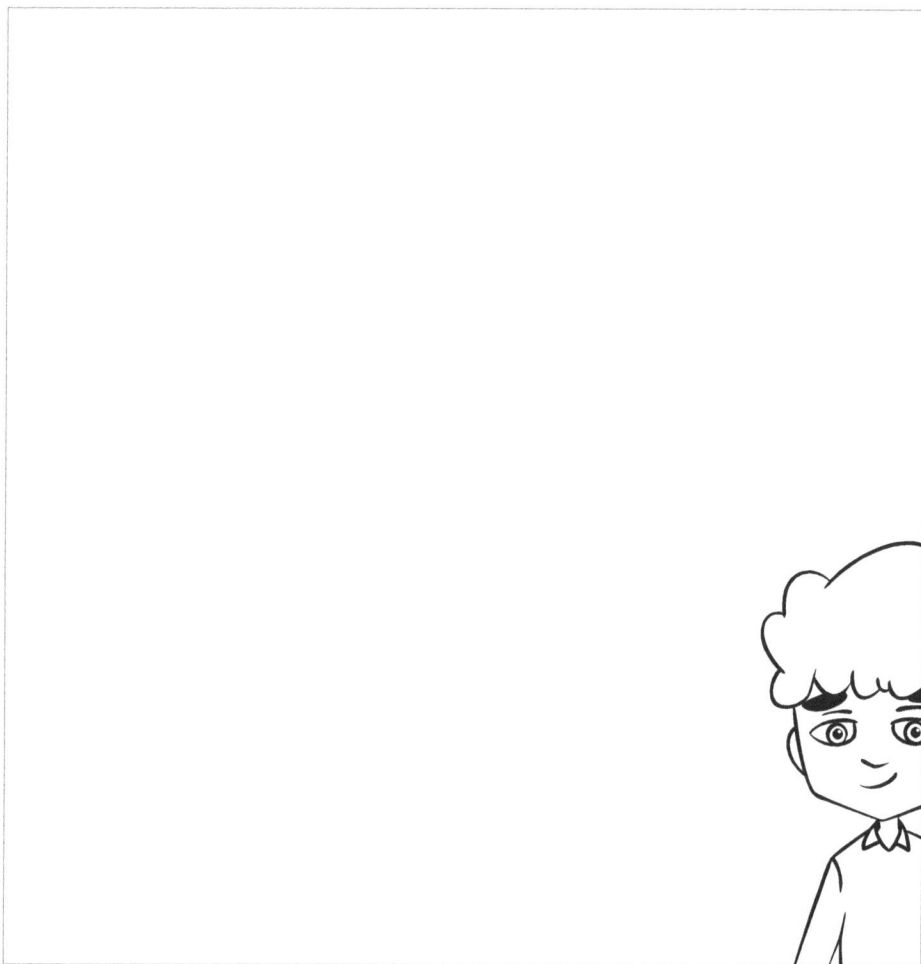

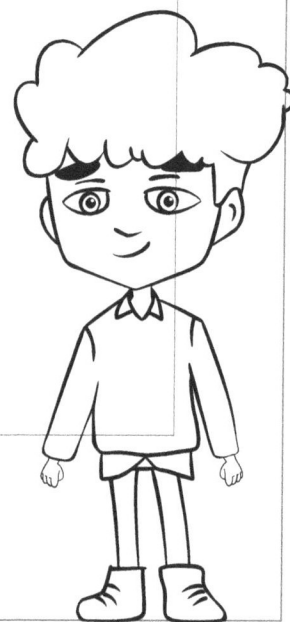

Date: _____

I can brush my teeth	I use a toothbrush
The dentist checks my teeth	My teeth are happy!

write a lil story about going to the dentist:

_____

_____

_____

Draw a picture of a happy tooth!

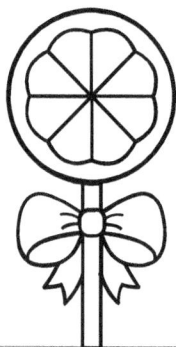

Draw a picture of dental floss:

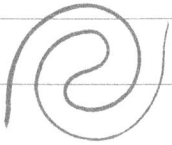

Draw a picture of the dental office:

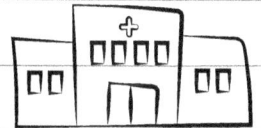

Draw a picture of the dental hygienist:

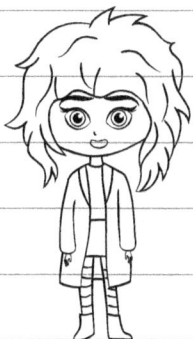

Date: _____

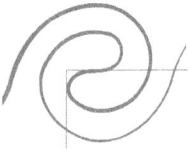

I will Floss my teeth everyday

Did I eat alot of sugar today?

How do my teeth feel today?

I will use mouthwash everyday

Write a lil story about your teeth:

_____

_____

_____

_____

Date: _____

My Next Dental Cleaning Will Be:

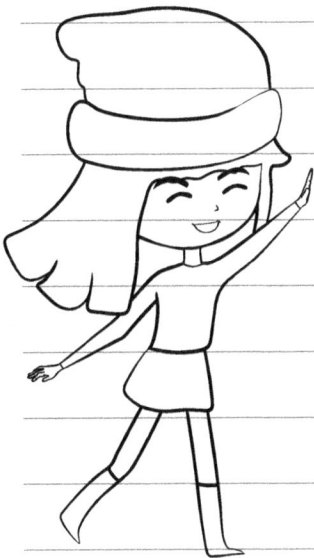

Write a note of thanks to the tooth fairy:

My tooth came out on this date

Write the amount the tooth fairy left under your pillow

Practice Writing:

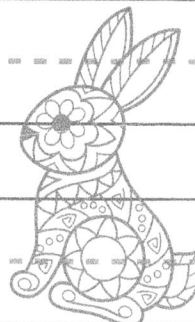

I have happy teeth

I love to brush my teeth

I love to floss my teeth

tooth

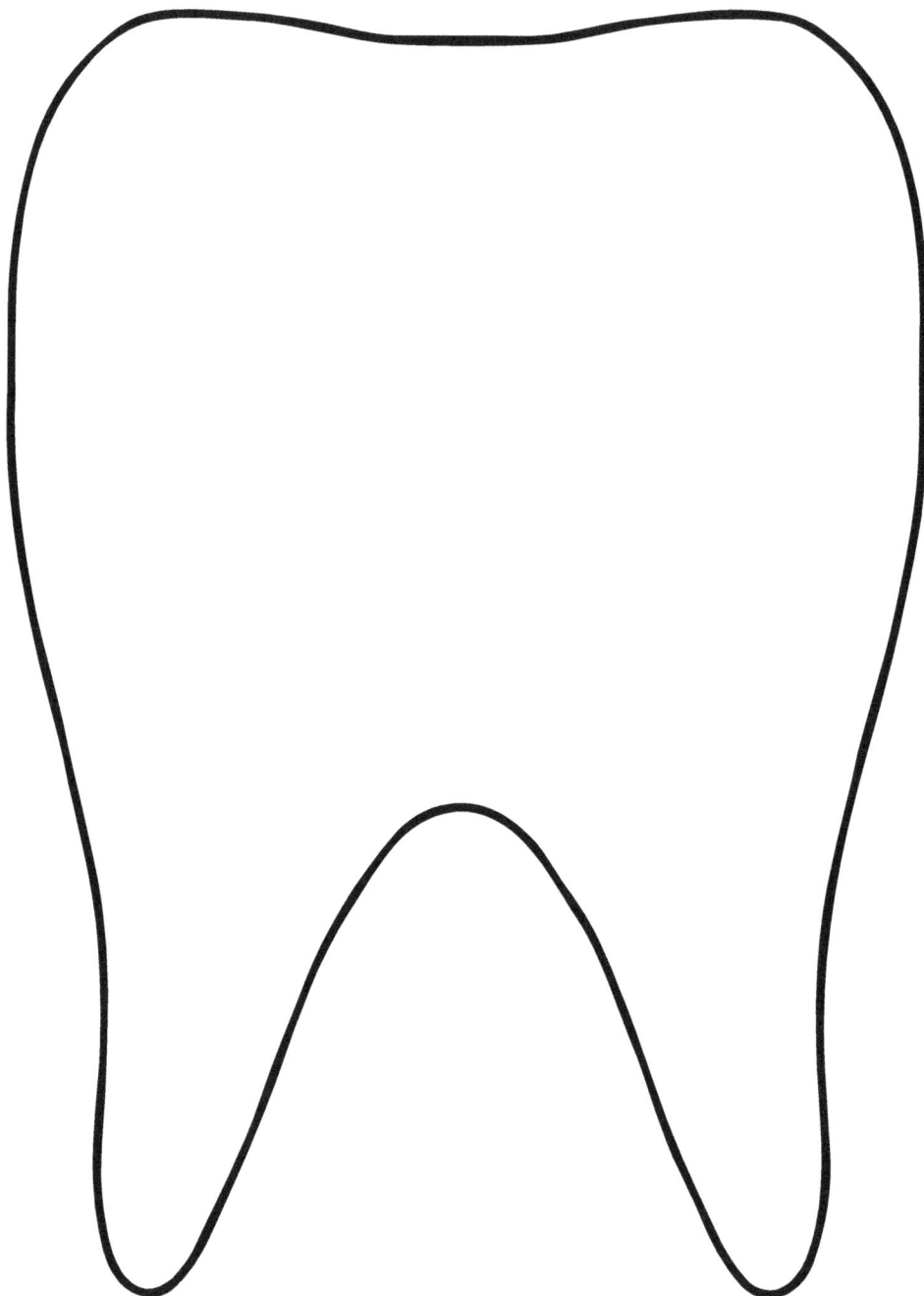

tooth x-ray

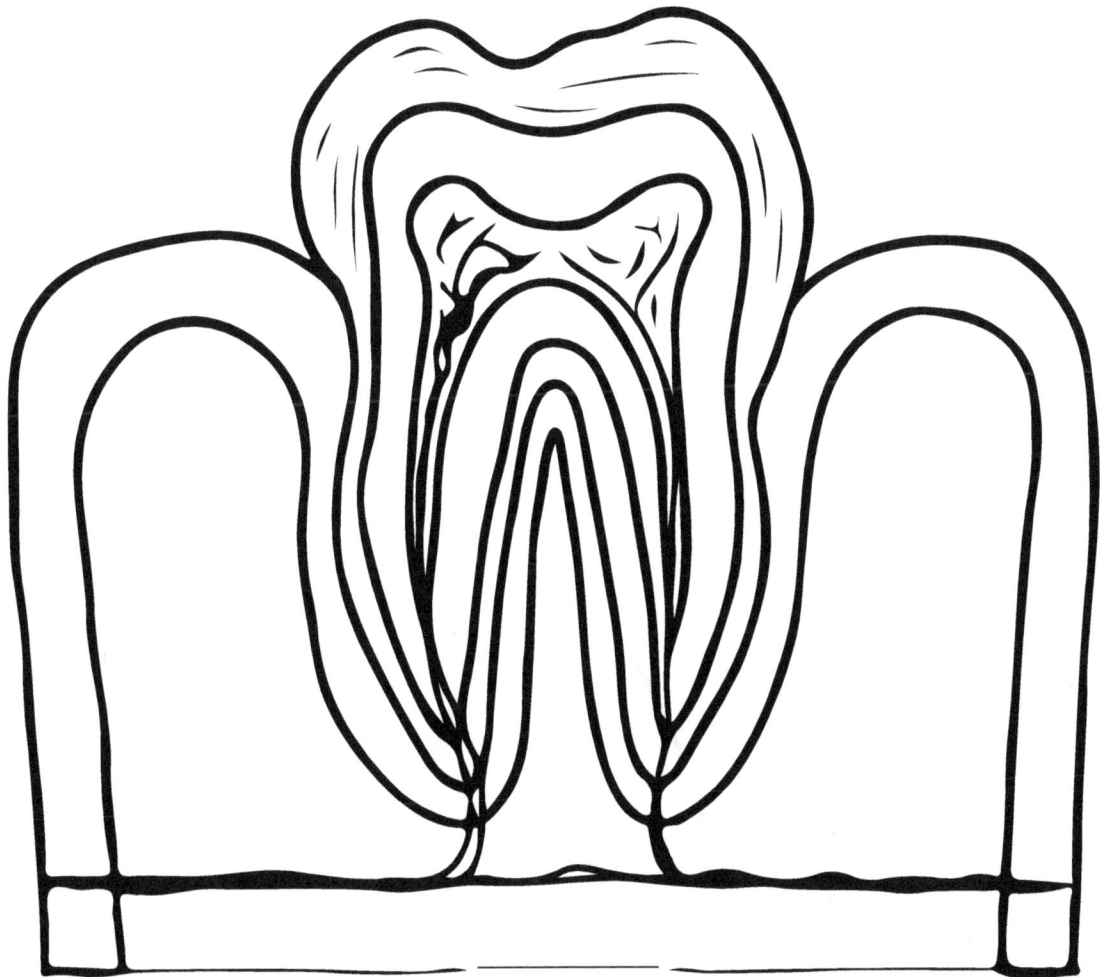

cavity

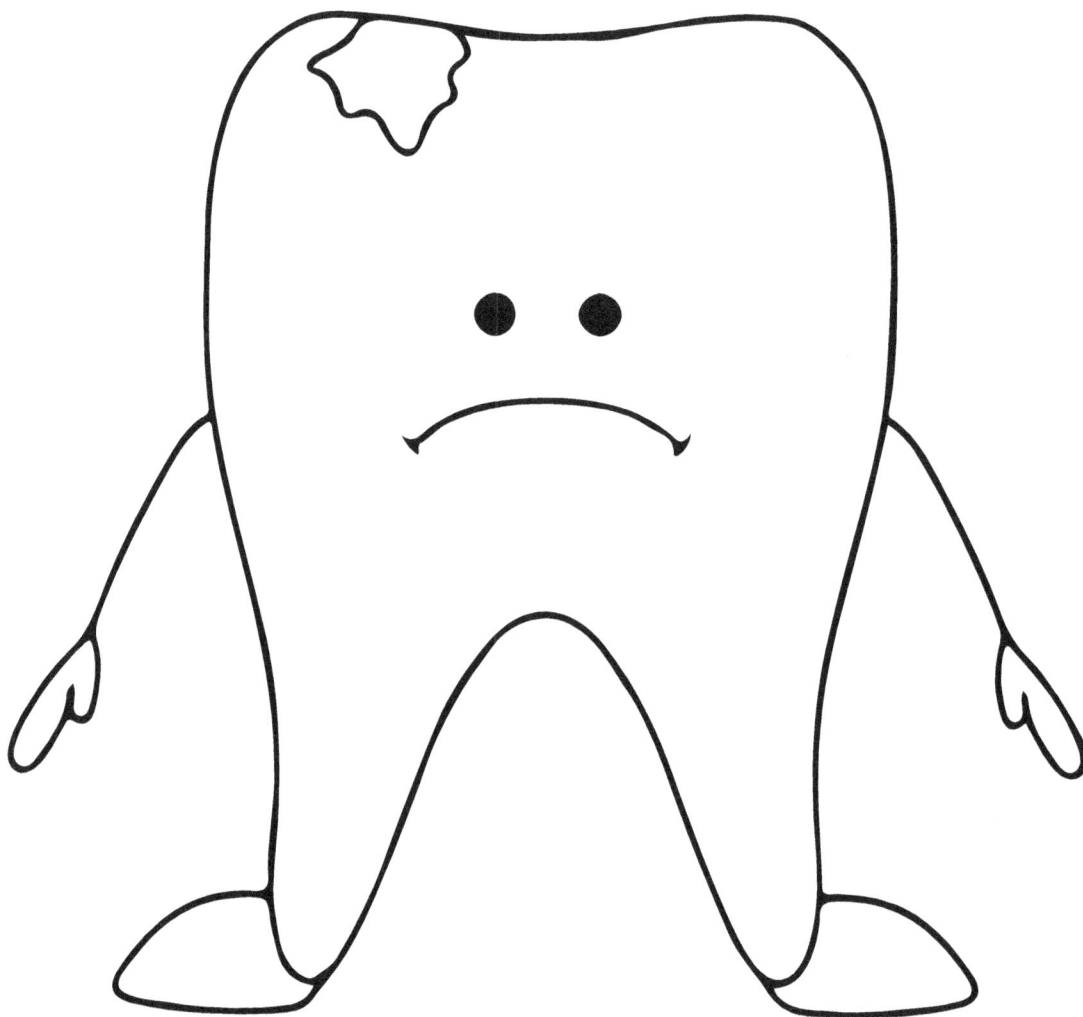

check-up

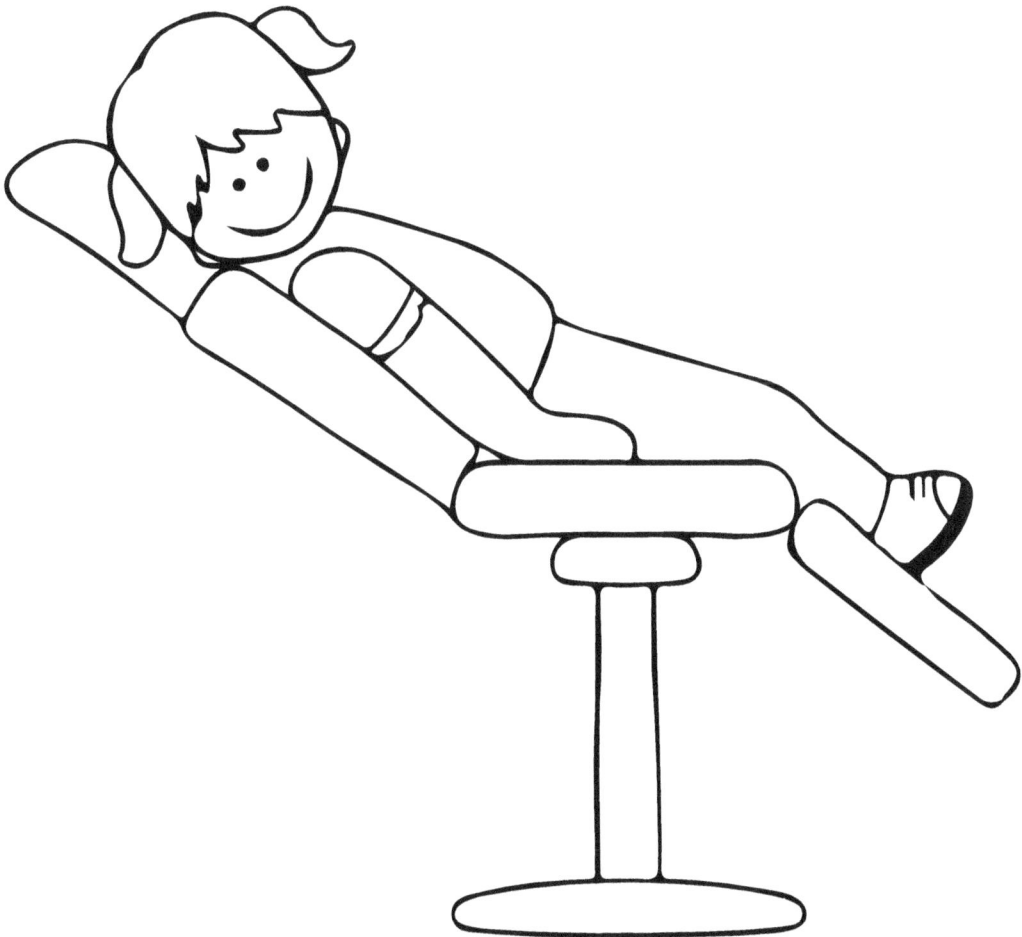

Tooth Fairy

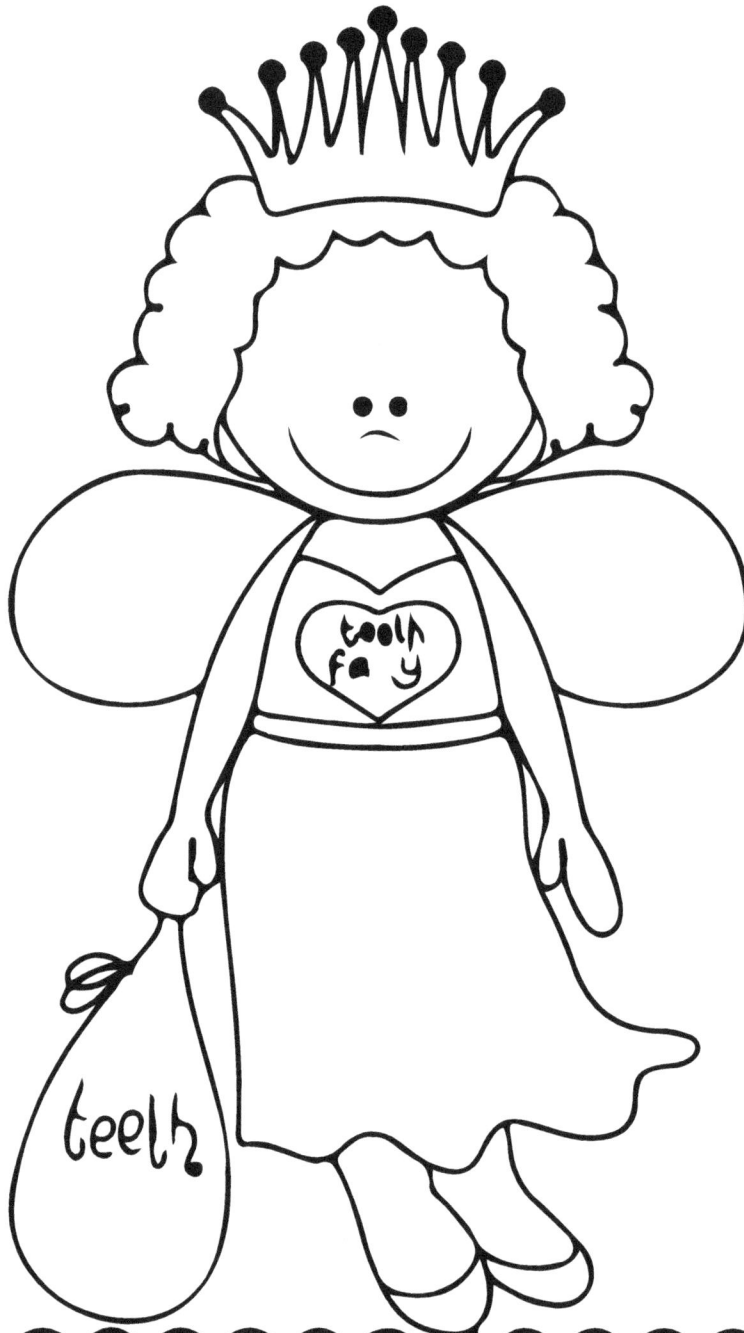

dentist

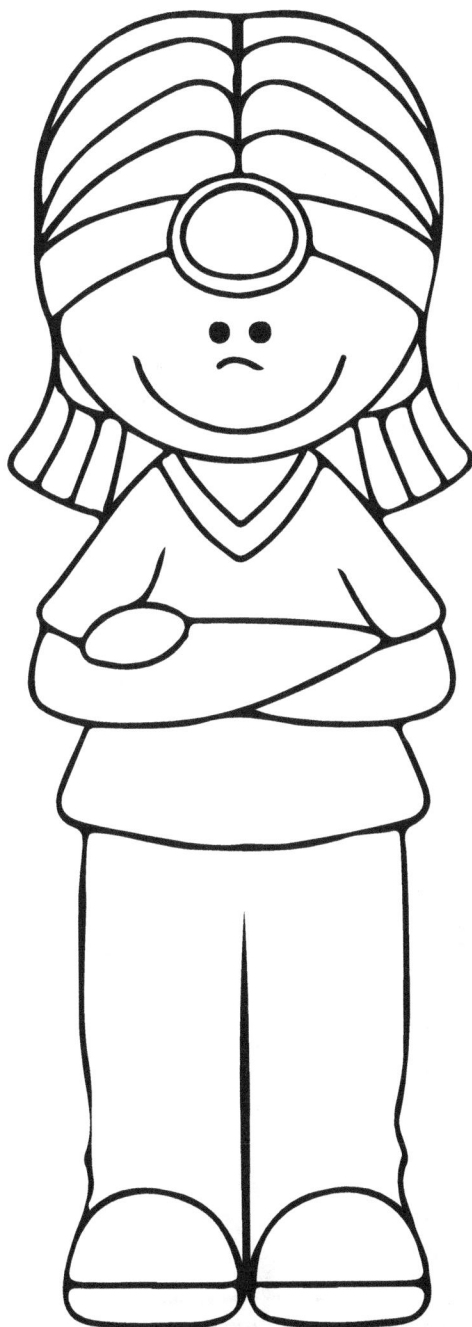

dentist

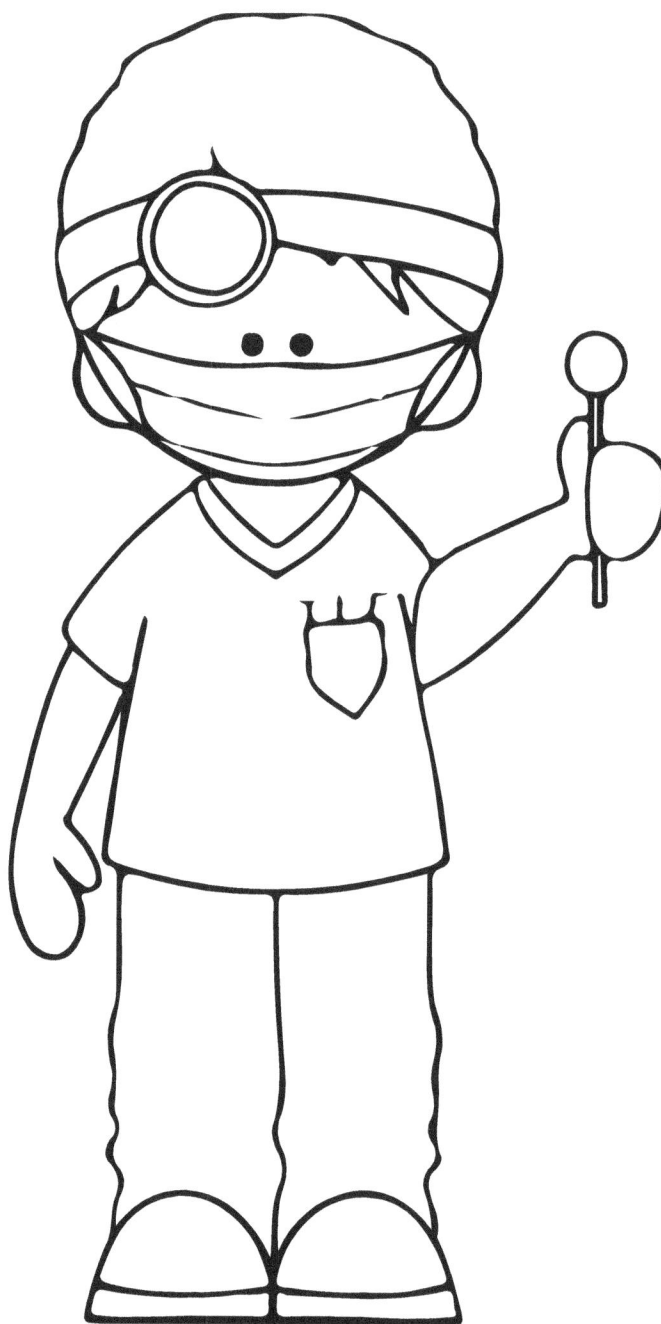

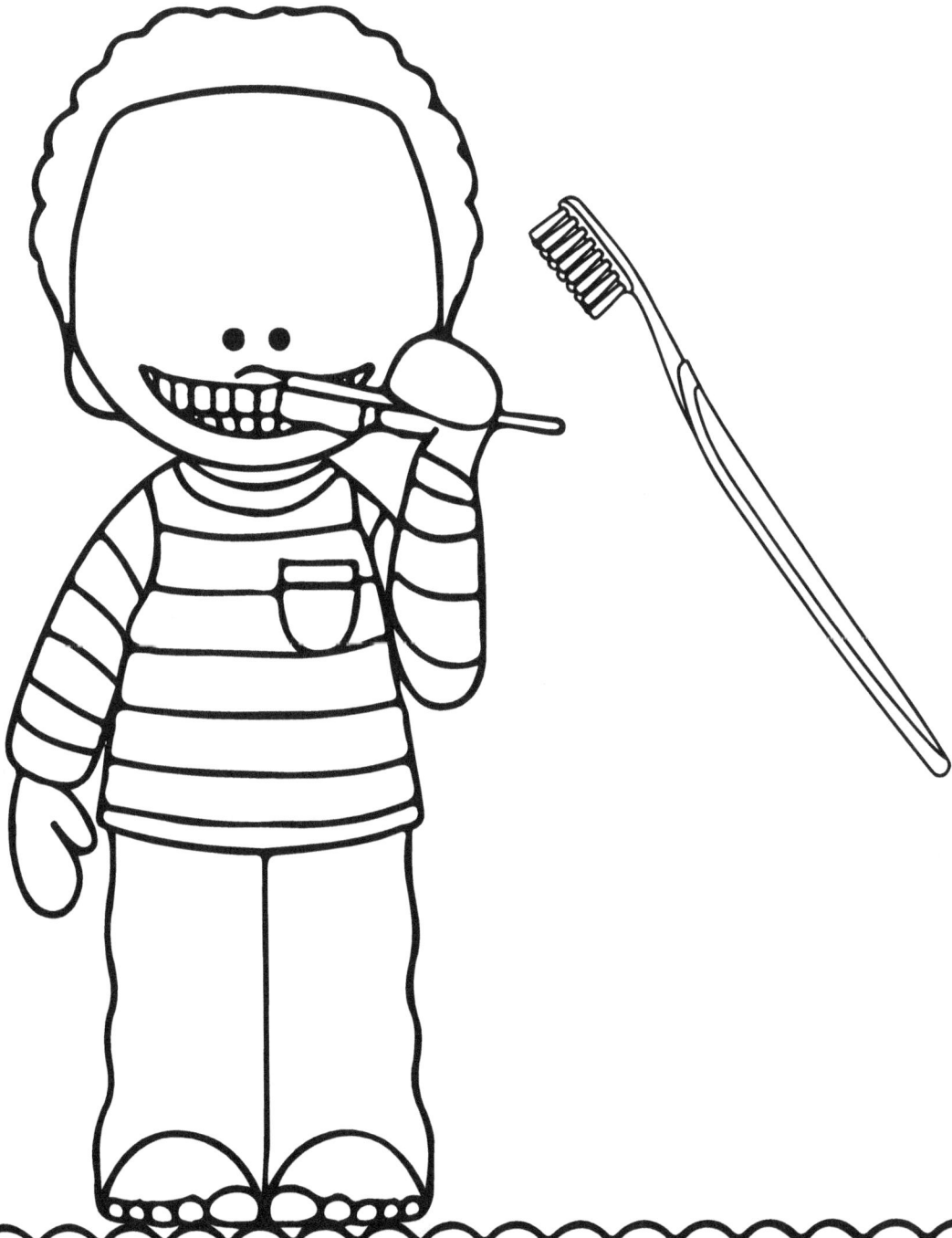

brush

brush

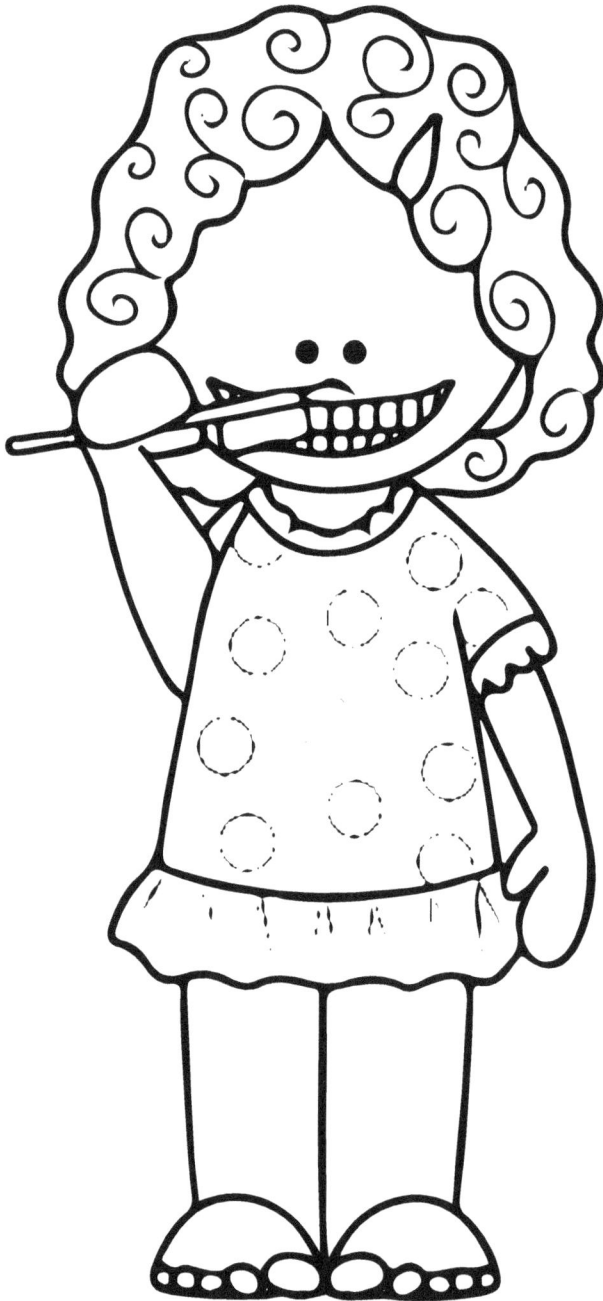
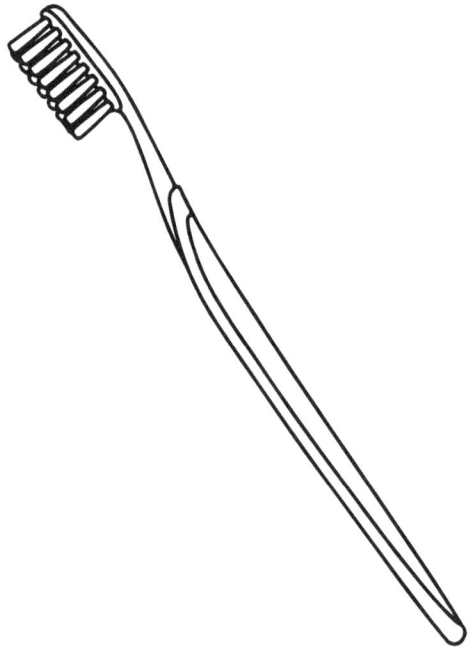

floss

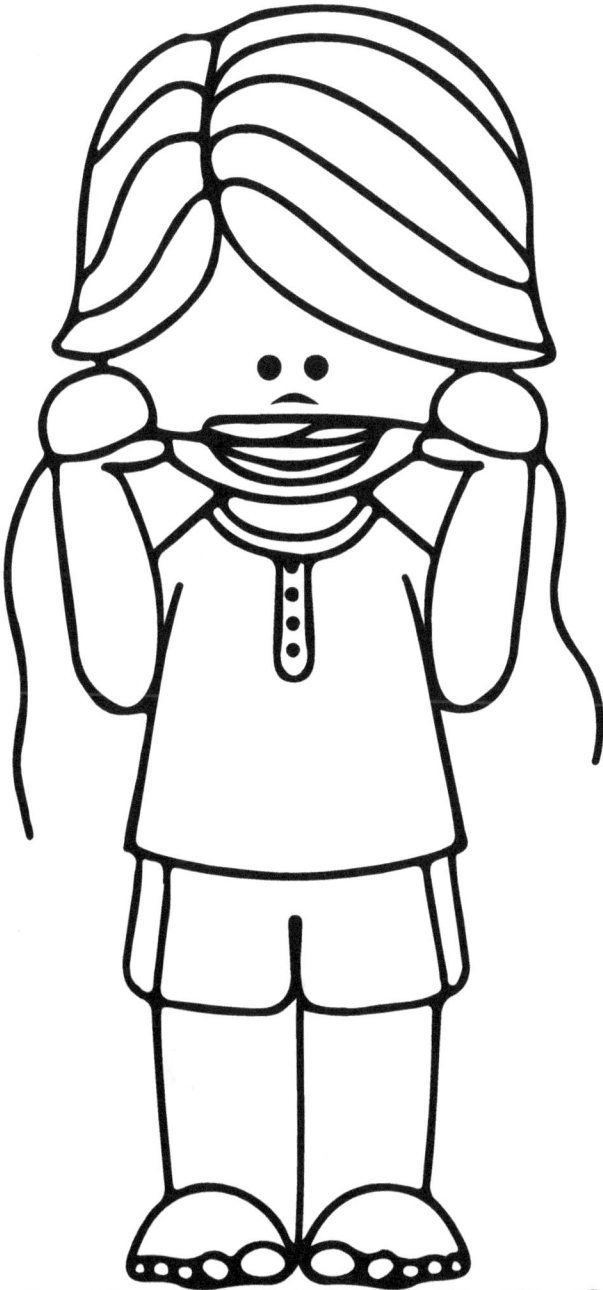

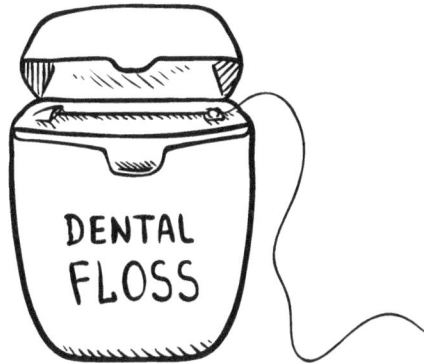

DENTAL
FLOSS

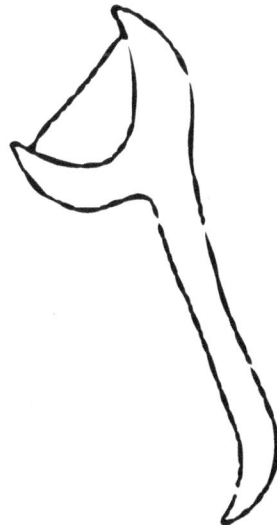

Color. Match.

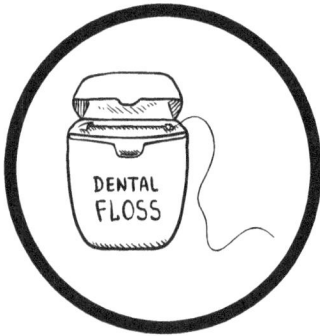

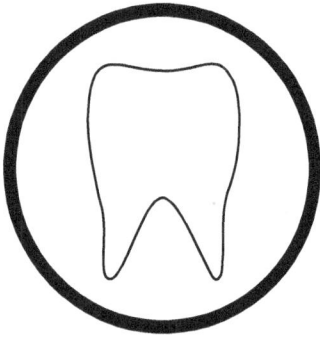

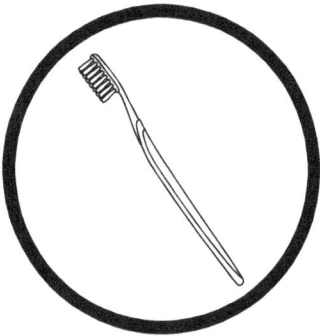

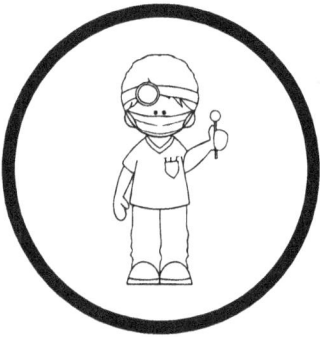

tooth

floss

dentist

toothbrush

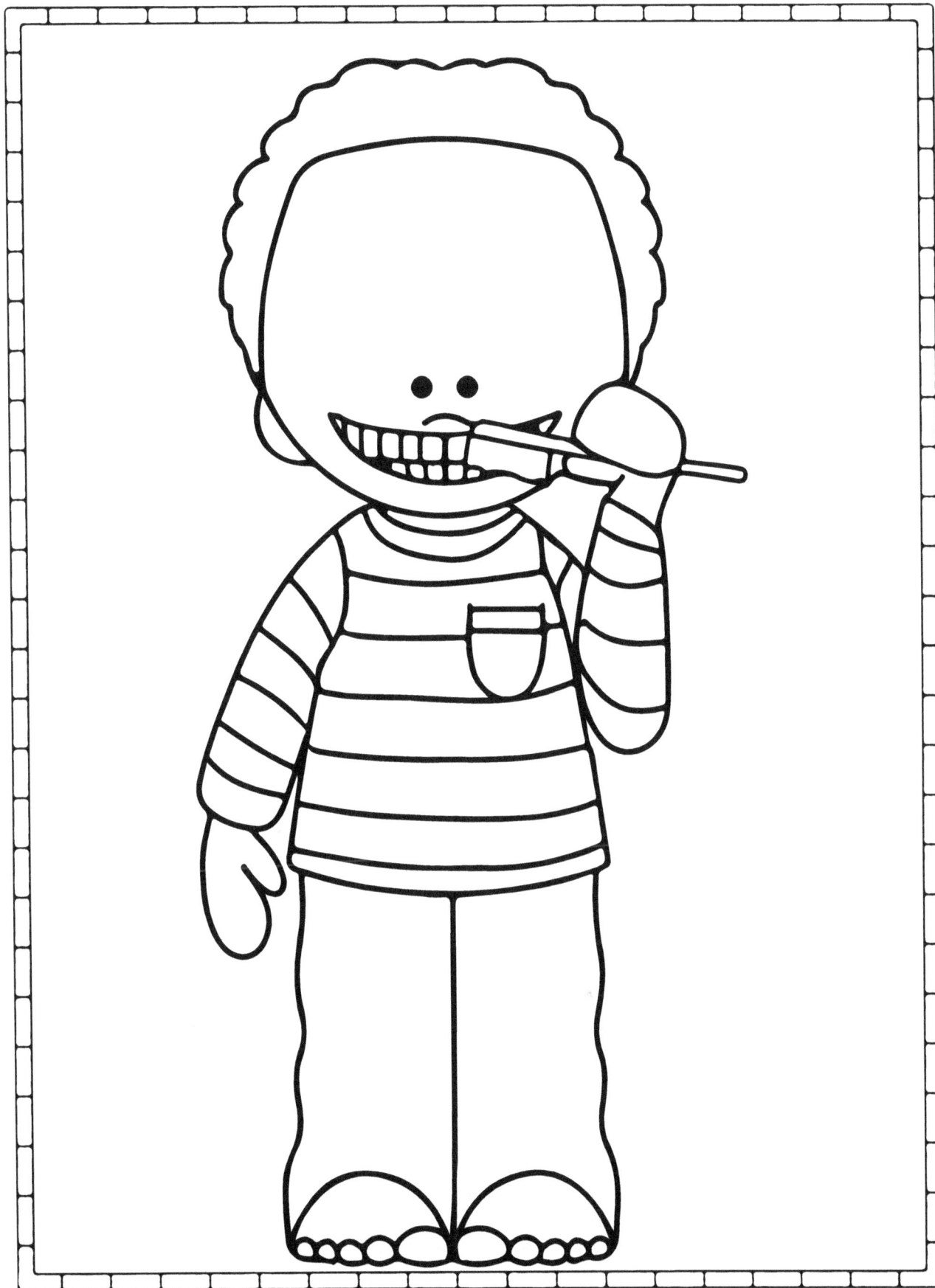

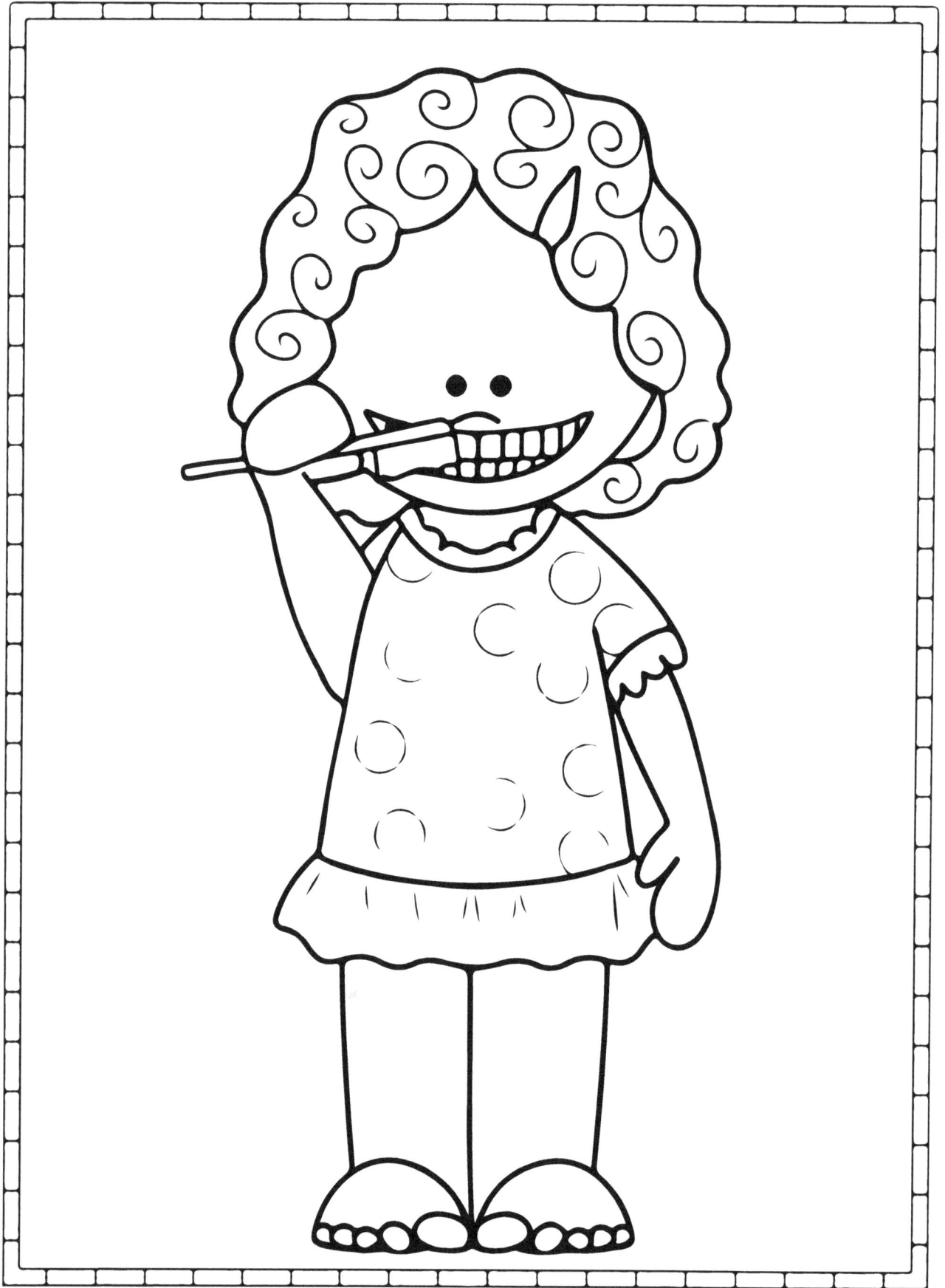

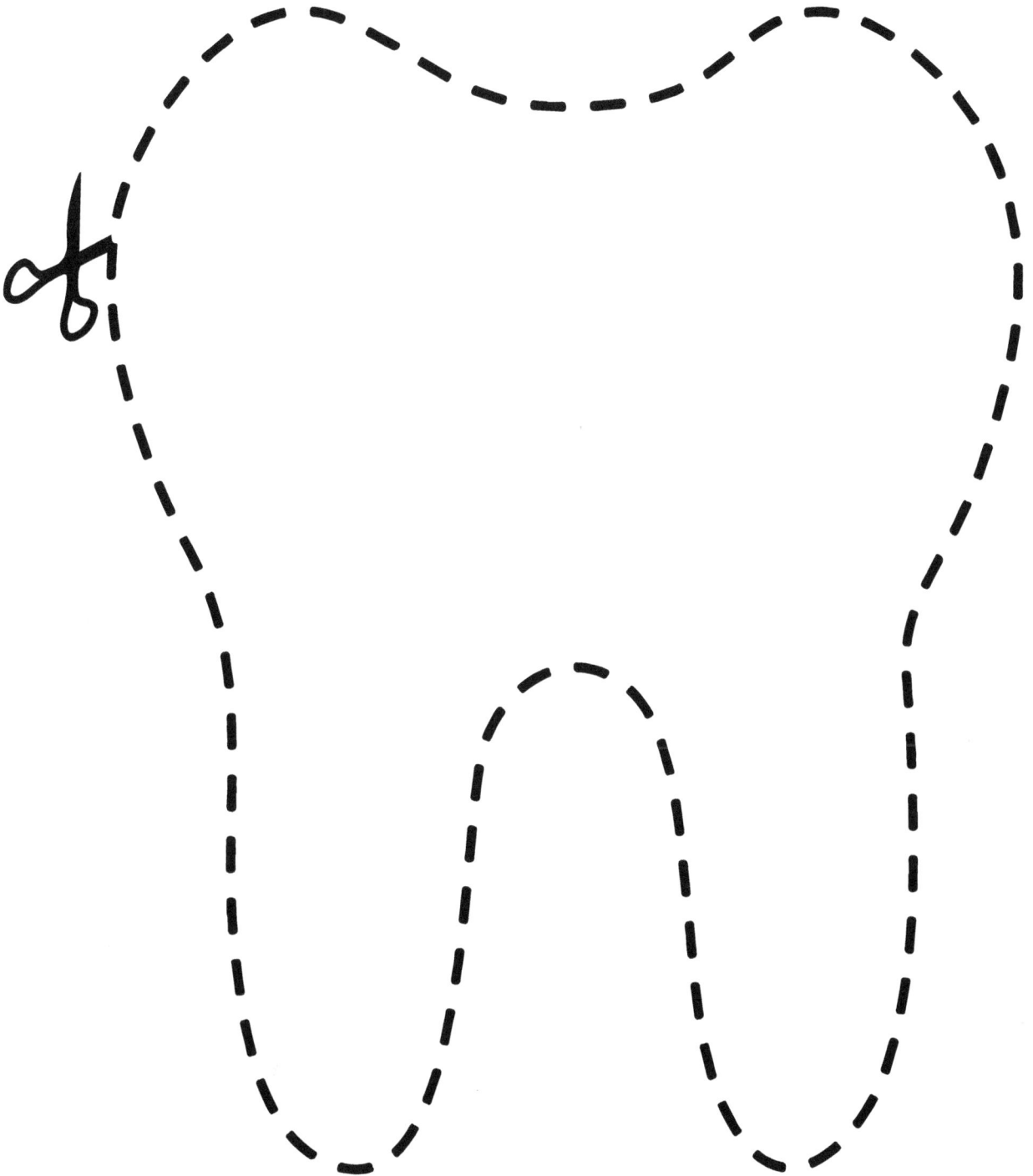

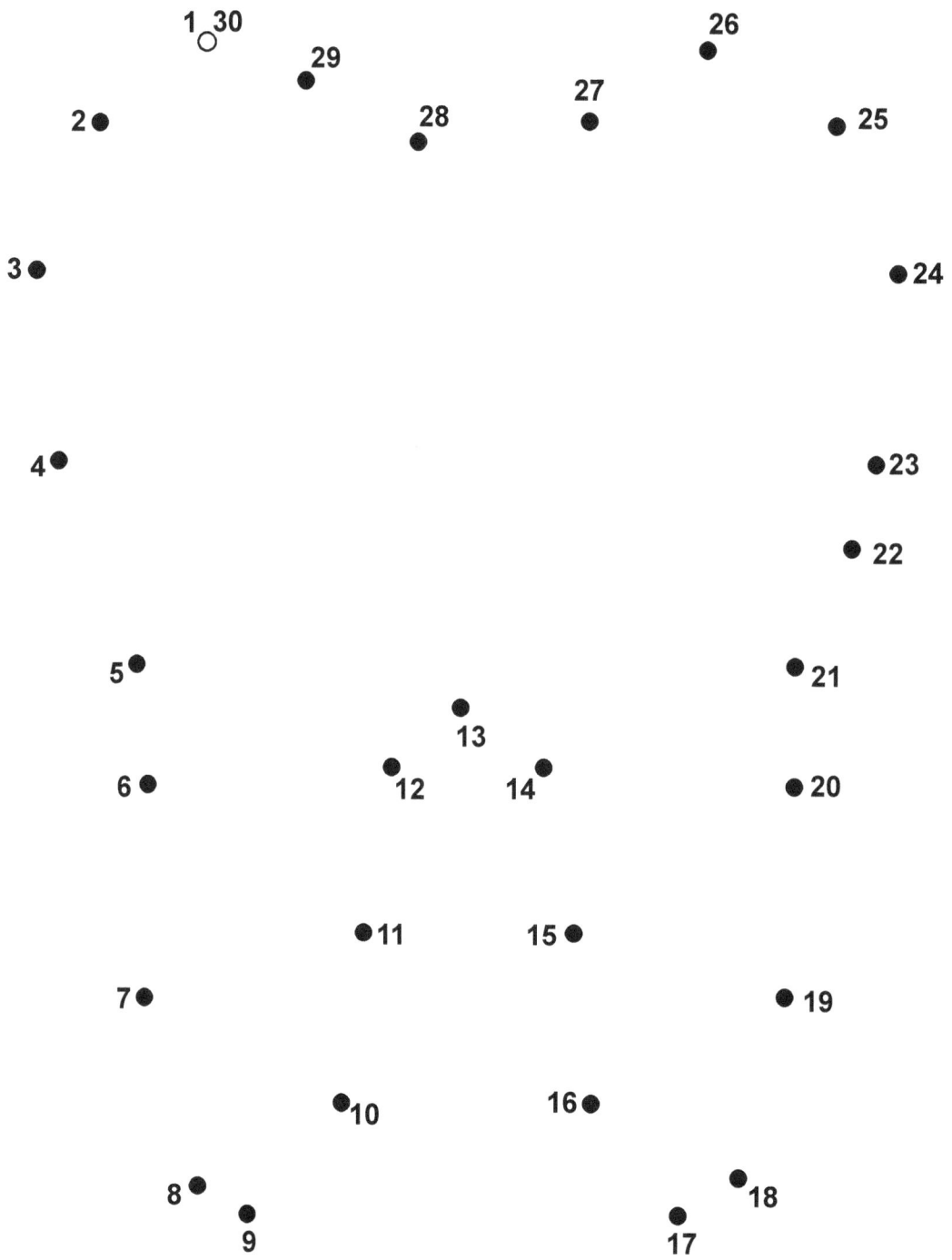

1 30
29
2
28
27
26
25
3
24
4
23
22
5
13
21
12 14
6
20
11 15
7
19
10 16
8
18
9 17

Draw a picture of a tooth:

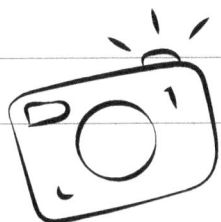

Draw a picture of your dentist

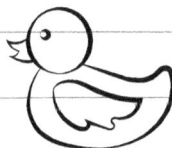

Draw a picture of your toothbrush:

Draw a picture of the tooth fairy:

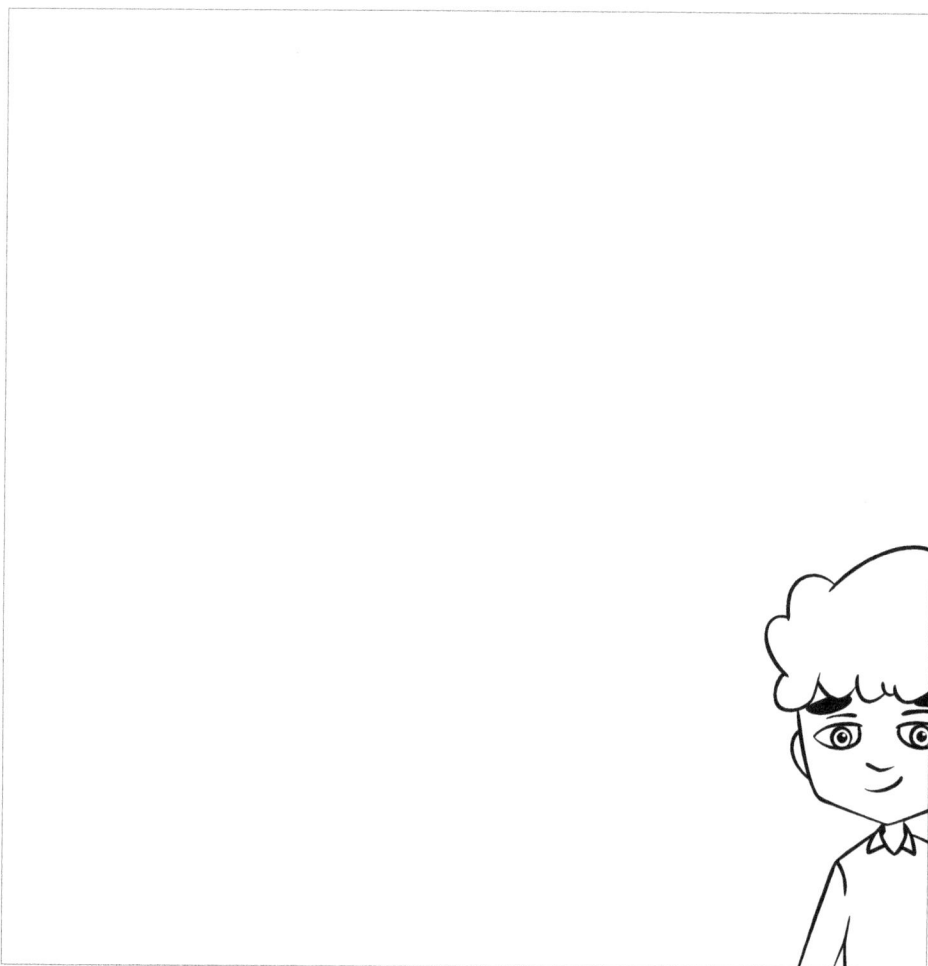

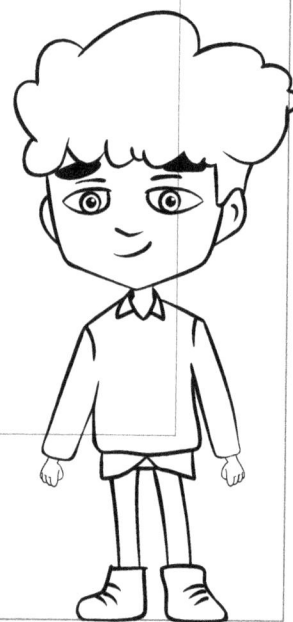

Date: _____

I can brush
my teeth

I use a
toothbrush

The dentist
checks my
teeth

My teeth
are
happy!

write a lil story about going to the dentist:

Draw a picture of a happy tooth!

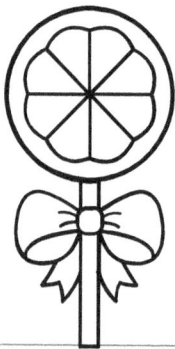

Draw a picture of dental floss:

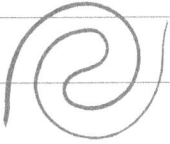

Draw a picture of the dental office:

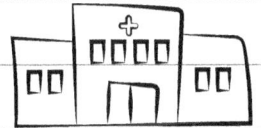

Draw a picture of the dental hygienist:

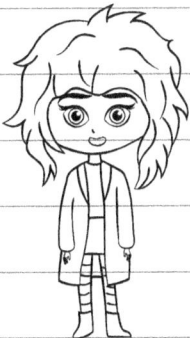

Date: _____

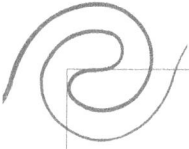

I will Floss my
teeth
everyday

Did I eat
alot of
sugar today?

How do
my teeth
feel today?

I will use
mouthwash
everyday

Write a lil story about your teeth:
_____
_____
_____
_____

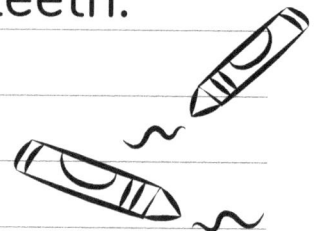

Date: _____

My Next Dental Cleaning Will Be:

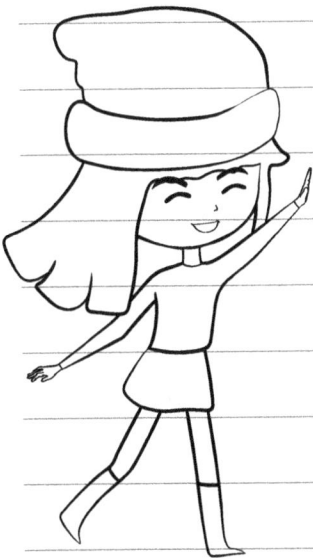

_____
_____
_____
_____
_____
_____
_____
_____
_____
_____

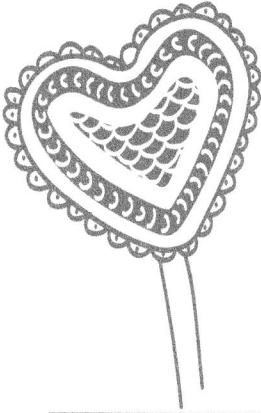

Write a note of thanks to the tooth fairy:

My tooth came out on this date

Write the amount the tooth fairy left under your pillow

Practice Writing:

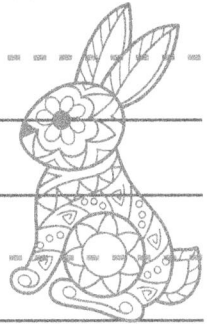

I have happy teeth

I love to brush my teeth

I love to floss my teeth

tooth

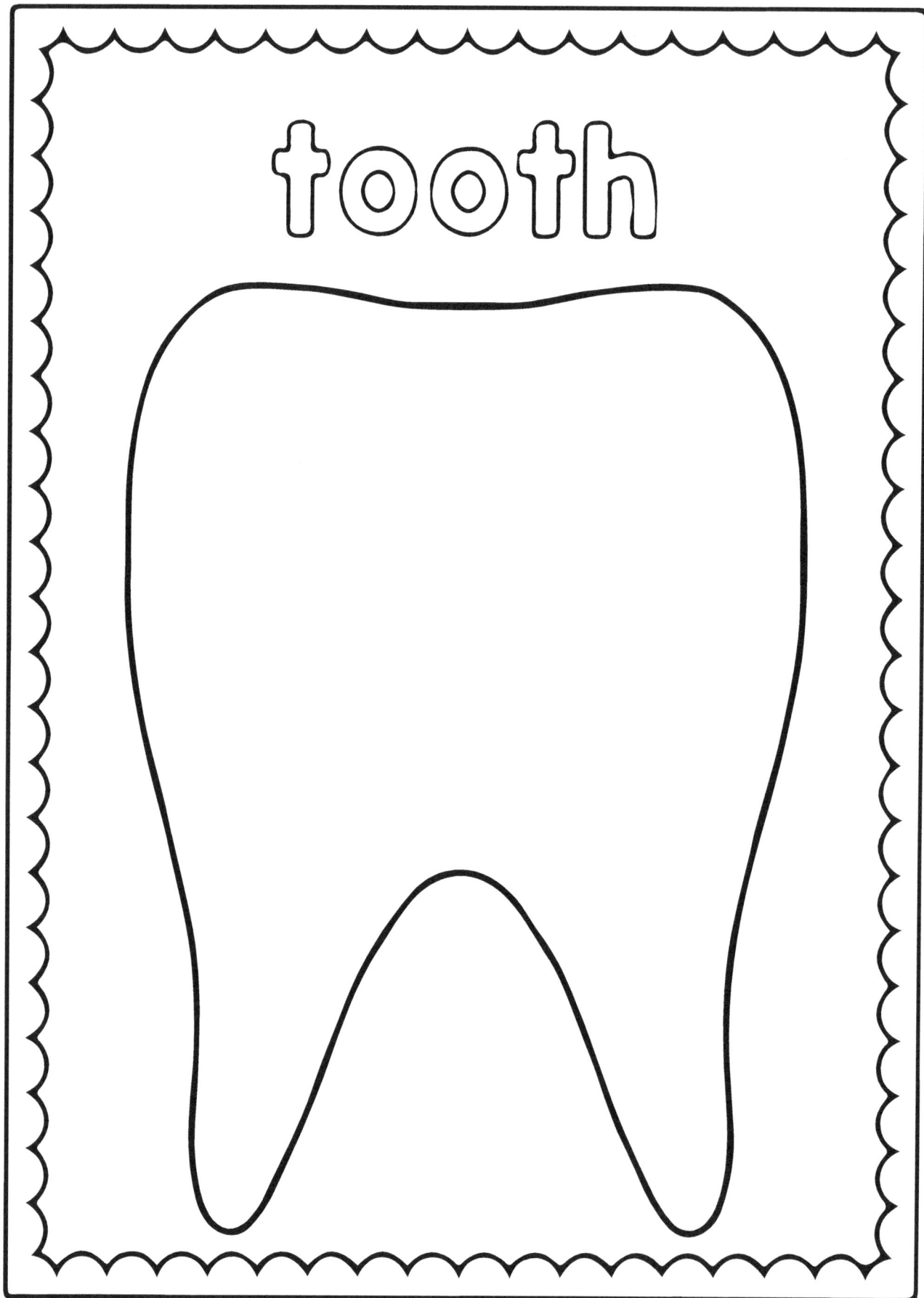

tooth x-ray

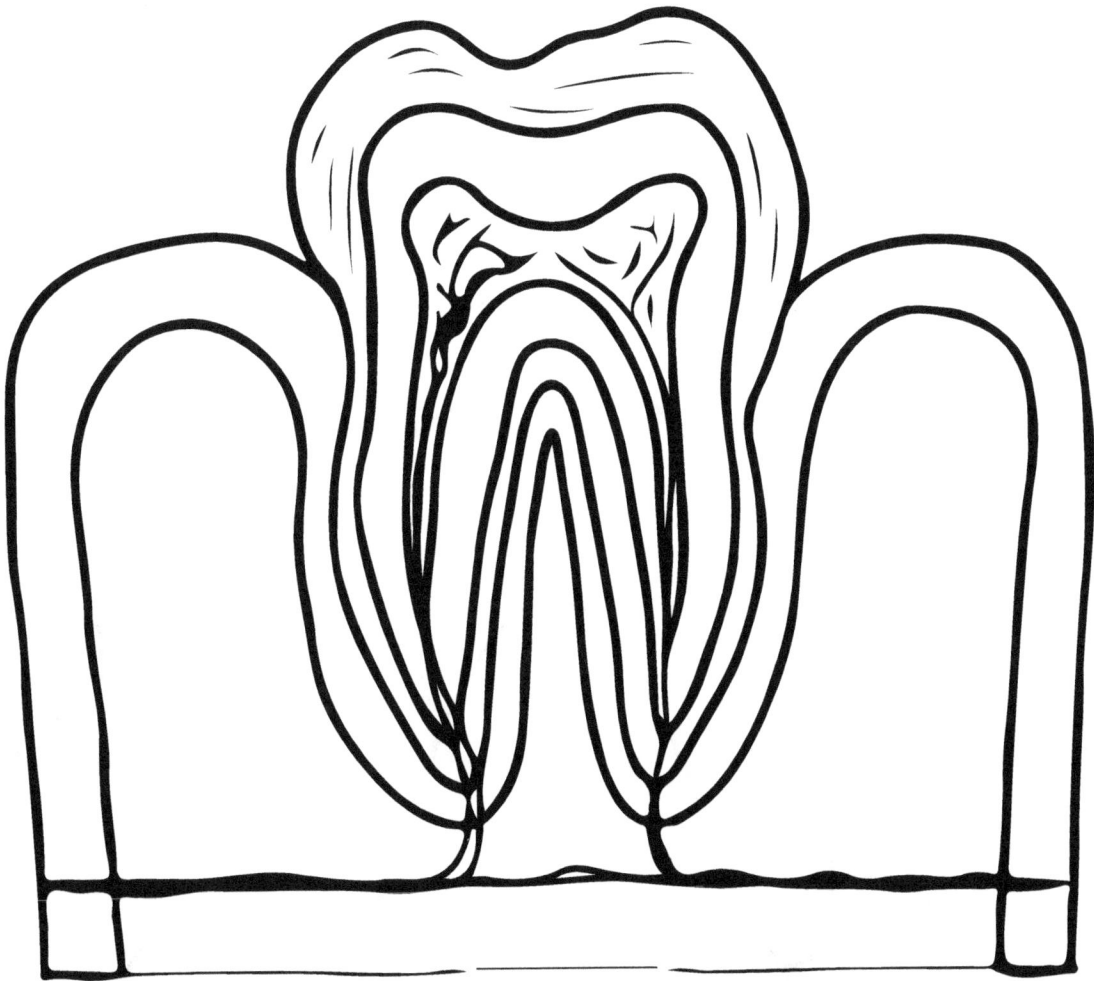

cavity

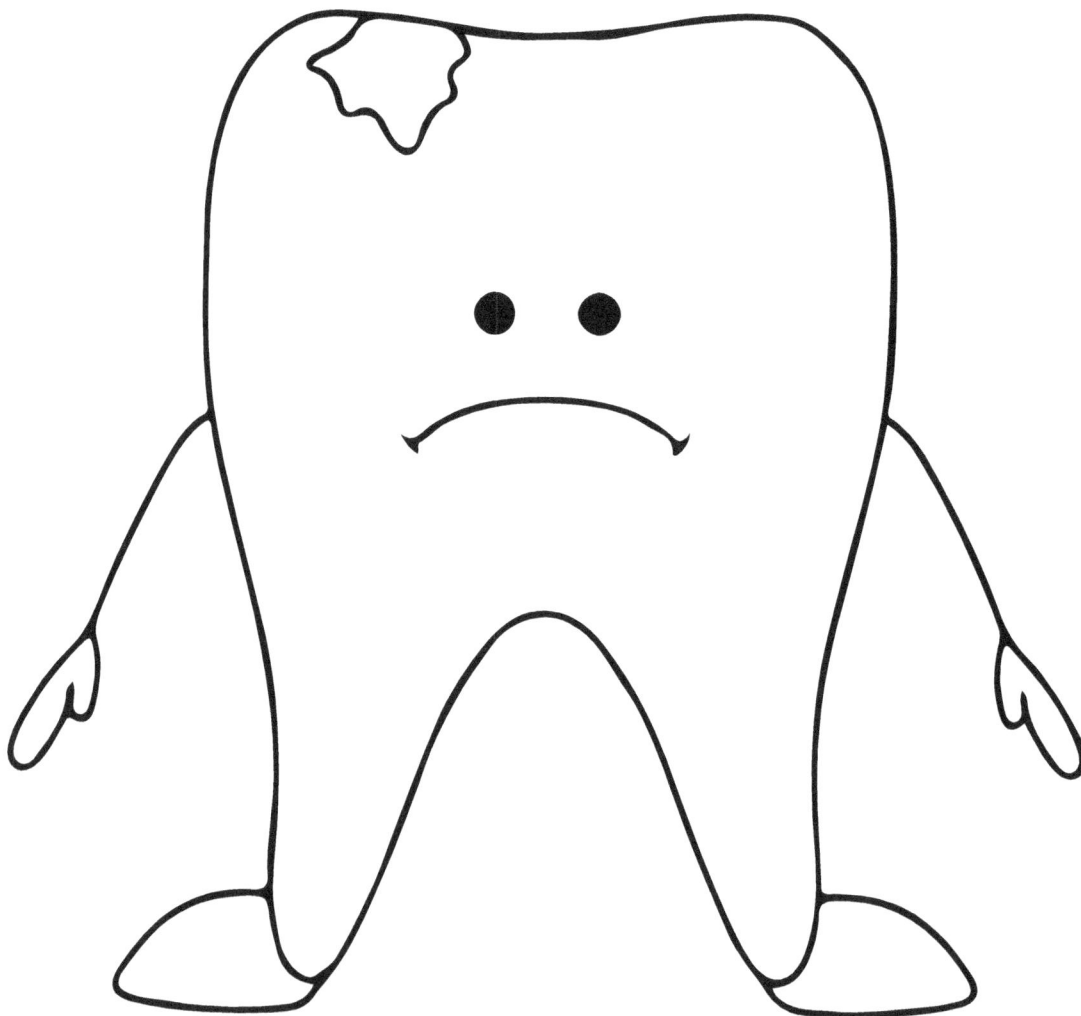

www.ingramcontent.com/pod-product-compliance
Lightning Source LLC
Chambersburg PA
CBHW081147020426
42333CB00021B/2695